RENAL RESILIENCE:

UNDERSTANDING AND CONQUERING KIDNEY STONES

I0454229

DR. MELISSA P. NELSON

Table of contents

PREFACE

In the intricate tapestry of human health, our bodies navigate a delicate balance, and at times, confront formidable challenges. Among the intricate web of organs, the kidneys stand as resilient guardians, silently toiling to maintain equilibrium. However, their strength is tested when crystalline structures, known as kidney stones, emerge as formidable adversaries.

This book, "Renal Resilience: Understanding and Conquering Kidney Stones," is an exploration into the fascinating realm of renal health. Within these pages, we embark on a journey to unravel the complexities of kidney stones, seeking not only to understand their formation and impact but also to empower individuals with the knowledge to conquer this common yet often underestimated health concern.

The genesis of this endeavor lies in the recognition that kidney stones are more than mere mineral formations within our bodies; they represent a significant health challenge that demands our attention and understanding. By delving into the intricate details of kidney stone formation, risk factors, and preventive measures, this book strives to be a comprehensive guide for both the curious reader and those grappling with the reality of kidney stones.

As we navigate through the chapters, we will uncover the scientific nuances of renal physiology, explore the various types of kidney stones, and delve into the factors that contribute to their formation. Alongside this scientific journey, we will emphasize the importance of resilience—the inherent ability of our bodies to rebound from adversity. Renal resilience is not just about bouncing back from the challenges posed by kidney stones; it is about understanding, managing, and ultimately conquering them.

To enhance the reader's experience, real-life stories and experiences will be woven into the narrative, providing a human touch to the scientific discourse. Moreover, the book will offer practical insights into lifestyle modifications, dietary choices, and medical interventions that can pave the way towards renal resilience.

My hope is that "Renal Resilience" serves as a beacon of knowledge and empowerment, offering readers the tools they need to navigate the intricate landscape of kidney health. Whether you are seeking preventive measures, dealing with the aftermath of kidney stones, or simply curious about the inner workings of your body, this book aspires to be your guide, providing both clarity and inspiration.

As we embark on this exploration together, let us unravel the mysteries of renal resilience, fostering a deeper understanding of our bodies and empowering ourselves to conquer the challenges that may arise along our health journey.

CHAPTER 1: INTRODUCTION

The human body is a marvel of intricate design, and nestled within its core are the kidneys, unsung heroes diligently performing the crucial task of maintaining balance. Yet, this equilibrium is disrupted when the seemingly innocuous process of crystalline formation transforms into a formidable health challenge: kidney stones.

Personal Motivation for Writing

As I embark on this exploration of renal resilience, my personal motivation stems from a deep-seated conviction that knowledge is the first step toward empowerment. Having witnessed the impact of kidney stones on individuals firsthand, whether through my professional encounters as a healthcare provider or in the lives of friends and family, I felt compelled to demystify the complexities surrounding this common ailment.

This book is not merely a compilation of scientific facts; it is a product of a fervent desire to empower readers with the insights needed to understand, manage, and conquer the challenges posed by kidney stones. Through shared experiences, practical advice, and a compassionate narrative, I aim to create a bridge between the intricacies of renal health and the lived realities of those grappling with kidney stones.

The Prevalence and Impact of Kidney Stones

As we delve into the prevalence of kidney stones, it becomes evident that this is not an isolated concern but a widespread health issue affecting millions worldwide. The impact of kidney stones extends beyond the physical realm, influencing the daily lives, well-being, and overall health of those affected.

This chapter seeks to establish a foundation for our journey by exploring the prevalence of kidney stones in diverse populations and shedding light on the multifaceted impact they can have on individuals. By understanding the scope of the challenge, we pave the way for informed discussions on preventive measures, treatment options, and the overarching theme of renal resilience.

Join me as we unravel the layers of renal health, driven by a shared commitment to knowledge, empowerment, and ultimately, conquering the formidable presence of kidney stones in our lives.

CHAPTER 2: UNDERSTANDING KIDNEY STONES

In the intricate landscape of renal health, understanding the nature and formation of kidney stones is paramount. As we embark on this journey, we delve into the intricate mechanisms that give rise to these crystalline structures, demystifying the process for both the curious mind and those grappling with the consequences.

Formation and Composition

Formation of Kidney Stones:

The formation of kidney stones is a complex process influenced by various factors, including the concentration of substances in the urine, the pH of the urine, and the presence of substances that promote or inhibit crystal formation. The general process of kidney stone formation involves the following steps:

1. Supersaturation: Urine contains various substances, including salts, minerals, and chemicals. When the concentration of these substances becomes too high, the urine becomes supersaturated. This means that the urine contains more dissolved salts and minerals than it can hold in a liquid state.

2. Nucleation: Supersaturation can lead to the formation of tiny crystals, a process known as nucleation. These crystals can consist of calcium, oxalate, phosphate, uric acid, or other substances found in urine.

3. Crystal Growth: Once nucleation occurs, the crystals can grow larger over time. The crystals may aggregate and stick together, forming solid particles.

4. Crystal Aggregation: Crystals can stick to each other, forming larger aggregates. The size of these aggregates can range from small particles to larger stones.

5. Stone Formation: As these aggregates grow and accumulate, they can form into kidney stones. The stones can vary in size, and their composition depends on the specific minerals and substances present in the urine.

Composition of Kidney Stones:

The composition of kidney stones can vary, and different types of stones are associated with specific minerals and compounds. The four main types of kidney stones and their compositions are:

1. Calcium Oxalate Stones: These are the most common type of kidney stones and are primarily composed of calcium oxalate. High levels of oxalate in the urine, combined with calcium, can lead to the formation of these stones.

2. Calcium Phosphate Stones: These stones are composed of calcium phosphate. They may form in conditions with alkaline urine.

3. Uric Acid Stones: Elevated levels of uric acid in the urine can lead to the formation of uric acid stones. Conditions such as gout or certain metabolic disorders can contribute to the development of these stones.

4. Struvite Stones: These stones are composed of magnesium, ammonium, and phosphate. They often result from urinary tract infections and can grow quickly.

Understanding the composition of kidney stones is essential for determining the underlying causes and developing appropriate prevention and treatment strategies. Individuals who are prone to kidney stones may benefit from dietary changes, increased fluid intake, and medications to manage specific conditions that contribute to stone formation. If someone suspects they have kidney stones, it is important to seek medical attention for proper diagnosis and guidance on treatment options.

Types of Kidney Stones

Within the intricate realm of renal health, the formation of kidney stones manifests in a variety of types, each distinguished by its unique composition and characteristics. As we navigate the diverse landscape of these crystalline structures, understanding the nuances of each type becomes pivotal for effective prevention and treatment strategies.

- **Calcium Oxalate Stones:**
Preeminent among kidney stones, calcium oxalate stones constitute a substantial majority of cases. These stones form when there is an excess of calcium and oxalate in the urine, leading to the crystallization of these substances. Dietary choices, genetic factors, and certain medical conditions can contribute to the elevated levels of calcium and oxalate, laying the groundwork for the formation of these stones.

- **Uric Acid Stones:**
For individuals with heightened levels of uric acid in their urine, the risk of developing uric acid stones is

elevated. These stones are particularly prevalent in those with conditions such as gout, where the body produces an excess of uric acid. Dehydration and diets rich in purines, found in certain foods, can exacerbate uric acid stone formation.

- **Struvite Stones:**

Struvite stones, also known as infection stones, arise in the context of urinary tract infections. These stones are unique in their composition, typically comprising magnesium, ammonium, and phosphate. The presence of certain bacteria in the urinary tract promotes the formation of struvite stones. Their large size and potential to cause blockages make prompt diagnosis and intervention imperative.

- **Cystine Stones:**

Cystine stones are a rarity, emerging in individuals with cystinuria, a hereditary condition characterized by the excessive excretion of cystine—a type of amino acid—in the urine. Due to its low solubility, cystine readily forms crystals, which aggregate to create stones. Management of cystine stones often requires a multifaceted approach, addressing both dietary and medical aspects.

- **Other Rare Types:**

Beyond the aforementioned common types, there exist rarer forms of kidney stones, such as those stemming from medications, like indinavir, or associated with specific medical conditions. While less prevalent, these types underscore the diverse nature of kidney stone formation, necessitating tailored approaches for their prevention and treatment.

Navigating the intricacies of these kidney stone types is essential for a comprehensive understanding of renal health. In the subsequent chapters, we will delve deeper into the specific characteristics, risk factors, and management strategies associated with each type, providing a roadmap for those seeking to conquer the challenges posed by kidney stones.

CHAPTER 3: CAUSES AND RISK FACTORS

In the labyrinth of renal health, the emergence of kidney stones is often influenced by a myriad of factors. Understanding the causes and risk factors that contribute to the formation of these crystalline structures is pivotal in crafting strategies for prevention and management. In this chapter, we unravel the intricate web of elements that heighten the likelihood of encountering the formidable challenge of kidney stones.

- **Dietary Influences: The Culinary Canvas of Renal Health**

Diet plays a pivotal role in the formation of kidney stones. High levels of oxalate-rich foods, such as beets, chocolate, and nuts, can contribute to calcium oxalate stones. Similarly, diets rich in purines, found in organ meats and certain seafood, can elevate uric acid levels, fostering the development of uric acid stones. This section explores the delicate balance between culinary choices and renal health, offering insights into dietary adjustments that can mitigate the risk of kidney stone formation.

- **Hydration and Dehydration: The Fluid Dynamics of Kidney Stones**

In the intricate dance of renal resilience, hydration emerges as a crucial partner. Insufficient fluid intake can concentrate minerals in the urine, laying the groundwork for the crystallization process. Conversely, maintaining optimal hydration levels can dilute urine and discourage the formation of kidney stones. This segment delves into the delicate fluid dynamics that influence renal health and offers practical tips for promoting adequate hydration.

- **Genetic Predispositions: Unlocking the Code of Renal Resilience**

The genetic landscape plays a significant role in an individual's susceptibility to kidney stones. Certain inherited conditions, such as cystinuria, can predispose individuals to specific types of stones. This section explores the intricate interplay between genetics and renal health, shedding light on the hereditary factors that contribute to the formation of kidney stones.

- **Medical Conditions and Interventions: Beyond the Stones**

Certain medical conditions, including urinary tract infections, metabolic disorders, and inflammatory bowel diseases, can create an environment conducive to kidney stone formation. Additionally, the use of certain medications can influence the composition of urine, potentially leading to stone development. This segment investigates the broader medical context within which kidney stones may arise, offering a holistic perspective on their causative factors.

- **Lifestyle Factors: The Tapestry of Renal Resilience**

Beyond diet and genetics, lifestyle factors such as obesity, sedentary habits, and geographical location can influence the risk of kidney stones. This section explores the multifaceted tapestry of lifestyle choices, providing insights into how modifying certain behaviors can contribute to renal resilience and diminish the likelihood of encountering kidney stones.

As we unravel the causes and risk factors associated with kidney stones, let us embark on a journey of awareness and proactive engagement. By understanding the intricate interplay of these elements, we pave the way for informed decisions that fortify our renal resilience and empower us to conquer the challenges posed by kidney stones.

Dietary Contributors

In the intricate interplay of factors influencing kidney stone formation, dietary choices emerge as powerful contributors. The foods we consume play a pivotal role in shaping the mineral composition of urine, ultimately influencing the likelihood of crystalline structures taking form within the kidneys. This exploration into dietary contributors aims to unravel the complex relationship between what we eat and the resilience of our renal health.

- **Oxalate-Rich Foods: The Calcium Oxalate Conundrum**

A significant dietary contributor to the formation of calcium oxalate stones lies in the consumption of foods high in oxalate. Spinach, beets, nuts, chocolate, and certain grains are among the culprits. Oxalate, when combined with calcium, forms crystals that can aggregate and evolve into kidney stones. Understanding the oxalate content of various foods is essential for individuals aiming to manage their risk of developing these common stones.

- **High-Purine Fare: Elevating Uric Acid Levels**

For those prone to uric acid stones, the purine content in certain foods takes center stage. Organ meats, shellfish, and certain types of fish are rich in purines, which, upon breakdown, can elevate uric acid levels in the body. This section unravels the connection between dietary purines and uric acid stone formation, providing insights into moderation and alternative dietary choices.

- ## Sodium and Calcium: The Balance of Minerals

While calcium is a critical component of kidney stone formation, paradoxically, both excess and insufficient intake can contribute to stone risk. This section explores the delicate balance required for optimal renal health. High dietary sodium can increase the excretion of calcium in the urine, potentially leading to the formation of calcium-containing stones. Understanding the nuanced relationship between sodium, calcium, and kidney stones is pivotal for dietary management.

- ## Fluid Intake: Nurturing Renal Resilience

A cornerstone of kidney stone prevention lies in maintaining adequate fluid intake. Dehydration concentrates minerals in the urine, creating an environment conducive to crystal formation. Conversely, optimal hydration helps dilute urine, reducing the risk of stone development. This segment explores the crucial role of fluid dynamics in renal health and offers practical guidance for individuals seeking to enhance their fluid intake.

- **Plant-Based Diets: A Double-Edged Sword**

While plant-based diets are often celebrated for their health benefits, certain plant foods can contribute to kidney stone formation. High-oxalate vegetables and legumes, such as sweet potatoes and lentils, may pose challenges for individuals predisposed to calcium oxalate stones. Navigating the nuances of plant-based diets requires an understanding of these potential contributors while still capitalizing on the overall health advantages of such dietary choices.

In the intricate tapestry of dietary contributors to kidney stone formation, knowledge becomes a potent ally. Armed with an understanding of the impact of specific foods on renal health, individuals can make informed dietary decisions that foster resilience and diminish the risk of encountering the formidable challenge of kidney stones.

Genetic Predispositions

Amidst the myriad factors influencing kidney stone formation, a significant role is played by our genetic makeup. The intricate dance of genes can confer predispositions that shape an individual's susceptibility to certain types of kidney stones. This exploration into genetic predispositions aims to unveil the inherited threads that weave into the complex fabric of renal health.

- **Cystinuria: The Amino Acid Imbalance**
Among the hereditary factors contributing to kidney stone formation, cystinuria stands out as a rare but impactful condition. This genetic disorder results in an abnormal excretion of the amino acid cystine in the urine. Cystine, being poorly soluble, readily forms crystals that aggregate into stones. Understanding the genetic underpinnings of cystinuria is essential for both diagnosis and the development of targeted management strategies.

- **Hypercalciuria: A Calcium Conundrum**

26

Genetic factors can also influence the reabsorption and excretion of calcium by the kidneys. Hypercalciuria, characterized by elevated levels of calcium in the urine, can predispose individuals to the formation of calcium-containing stones. This section explores the genetic components of calcium regulation and sheds light on how variations in these genetic factors may contribute to stone risk.

- **Hyperoxaluria: The Oxalate Dilemma**

Inherited conditions leading to increased oxalate production or impaired oxalate metabolism can contribute to hyperoxaluria. This elevated oxalate level in the urine heightens the risk of forming calcium oxalate stones. Genetic variations in enzymes involved in oxalate metabolism can impact an individual's predisposition to this particular type of kidney stone.

- **Familial Clustering: Shared Genetic Influences**

Studies suggest a familial tendency for kidney stone formation, indicating that shared genetic factors among family members may contribute to stone risk. While specific genes associated with this familial clustering are still under investigation, recognizing the genetic component in families with a history of kidney stones emphasizes the importance of genetic factors in renal health.

- **Genetic Variants and Metabolic Factors: The Intersection of Genes and Lifestyle**

Genetic predispositions interact with lifestyle factors, creating a dynamic interplay that influences an individual's susceptibility to kidney stones. This section delves into the intricate intersection of genetic variants and metabolic factors, emphasizing how understanding these relationships can guide personalized approaches to stone prevention.

As we unravel the genetic predispositions to kidney stone formation, we gain insights into the personalized nature of renal health. Recognizing the influence of inherited factors enables a proactive approach to managing and mitigating the risks associated with kidney stones, fostering a deeper understanding of the interplay between our genes and the resilience of our kidneys.

CHAPTER 4: RECOGNISING SYMPTOMS

In the intricate landscape of renal health, the presence of kidney stones often reveals itself through a symphony of subtle signals and, at times, more pronounced warnings. Recognizing these symptoms becomes paramount for early detection, timely intervention, and the effective management of the challenges posed by kidney stones. This chapter serves as a guide to deciphering the language of the body, shedding light on the varied symptoms that may herald the presence of kidney stones.

- **Fluctuating Pain: The Renal Melody**

A hallmark symptom of kidney stones is the fluctuating pain that can range from a dull ache to intense, stabbing sensations. This section explores the nuances of renal pain, including its location (often in the back or side) and the potential radiation to the lower abdomen and groin. Understanding the dynamic nature of this pain is crucial for distinguishing it from other sources and initiating timely diagnostic measures.

- **Hematuria: Traces of Blood in the Urine**

The presence of blood in the urine, known as hematuria, is a common indicator of kidney stones. Whether visible to the naked eye or detected through laboratory tests, hematuria underscores the potential impact of stones on the delicate tissues of the urinary tract. This segment delves into the significance of hematuria and its role as a key symptom in the diagnostic puzzle of kidney stones.

- **Urinary Changes: Unraveling the Clues**

Kidney stones can bring about changes in urinary patterns, manifesting as urgency, frequency, or difficulty in urination. Understanding these variations in urinary behavior is crucial for recognizing the potential influence of kidney stones on the normal functioning of the urinary system. This section explores the subtleties of urinary changes and their significance in the broader context of renal health.

- **Nausea and Vomiting: The Gastrointestinal Response**

Kidney stones can evoke a range of gastrointestinal symptoms, including nausea and vomiting. This segment explores the mechanisms by which kidney stones can trigger these responses and emphasizes the importance of recognizing these symptoms as potential indicators of underlying renal challenges.

- **Fever and Chills: Signs of Infection**

In certain cases, the presence of kidney stones can lead to urinary tract infections, accompanied by symptoms such as fever and chills. Recognizing these systemic signs is crucial, as they may point to complications associated with kidney stones that necessitate prompt medical attention.

- **Subtle Signs and Atypical Symptoms: The Mosaic of Presentation**

Beyond the more common symptoms, kidney stones can occasionally manifest in atypical ways. This section explores the mosaic of subtle signs, such as testicular pain, cloudy urine, or persistent bad breath, underscoring the diverse ways in which kidney stones can present themselves.

By delving into the diverse symphony of symptoms associated with kidney stones, this section aims to empower readers to recognize the early whispers of renal distress. Armed with this knowledge, individuals can take proactive steps towards diagnosis, intervention, and the pursuit of renal resilience in the face of the challenges posed by kidney stones.

Early Warning Signs

In the intricate landscape of renal health, kidney stones often unveil themselves through a series of early warning signs—subtle whispers that, when heeded, can prompt timely intervention and mitigate the impact of these crystalline formations. Recognizing these initial signals is pivotal for individuals to embark on a proactive journey toward understanding, managing, and conquering the challenges posed by kidney stones.

- **Mild, Intermittent Pain: The Prelude to Renal Discomfort**

One of the earliest warning signs of kidney stones is the presence of mild, intermittent pain. This discomfort often manifests as a dull ache in the back or side, signaling the initial stages of stone formation. Paying attention to these subtle twinges can serve as a crucial early indicator, prompting individuals to seek medical evaluation before the pain escalates.

- **Changes in Urination Patterns: The Whispers of the Urinary System**

Kidney stones can subtly influence urinary patterns, leading to changes in frequency, urgency, or the sensation of incomplete emptying. These alterations may be subtle initially but can serve as early warnings that merit attention. Recognizing deviations from one's normal urinary routine can pave the way for proactive investigation and potential early intervention.

- **Discolored Urine: The Palette of Hematuria**

An early indicator of kidney stones is the presence of discolored urine, often tinged with shades of pink or red. This is a result of hematuria, the occurrence of blood in the urine. While the discoloration may be subtle and intermittent, it serves as a noteworthy sign that warrants further investigation to uncover the underlying cause.

- **Nagging Nausea: Gastrointestinal Cues**

Before nausea evolves into a pronounced symptom, it may present as a subtle, nagging sensation. Kidney stones can trigger gastrointestinal distress, and recognizing these early hints of nausea can prompt individuals to consider the possibility of renal involvement. Addressing these cues in their incipient stages may contribute to early diagnosis and management.

- **Urinary Odor and Cloudiness: Subtle Clues in the Stream**

Changes in the odor and clarity of urine can be subtle but significant indicators of renal distress. Kidney stones may influence the composition of urine, leading to subtle alterations in its appearance and smell. Recognizing these nuances can contribute to the early identification of kidney stones and guide individuals toward seeking medical advice.

- **Generalized Fatigue: A Systemic Response**
Kidney stones, even in their early stages, can induce a generalized feeling of fatigue. While fatigue is a nonspecific symptom, recognizing it in conjunction with other subtle signs may prompt individuals to consider the possibility of kidney stones as an underlying cause, initiating a proactive approach to investigation and management.

By attuning themselves to these early warning signs, individuals can foster a proactive mindset toward their renal health. These subtle whispers, when deciphered and heeded, empower individuals to seek timely medical attention, unravel the mysteries of kidney stones, and embark on a journey towards resilience and conquering the challenges that may lie ahead.

When to Seek Medical Attention

In the intricate landscape of renal health, understanding when to seek medical attention is paramount, particularly when kidney stones cast their shadow over one's well-being. Timely intervention can make the difference between managing discomfort and preventing potential complications. This guide outlines the pivotal moments when individuals should heed the call for medical assistance in the context of kidney stones.

- **Persistent or Intense Pain: The Urgency of Discomfort**

Persistent or intense pain in the back, side, or lower abdomen is a compelling signal to seek medical attention. While mild discomfort may be an early warning, unrelenting or severe pain may indicate a larger stone or potential blockage. Prompt evaluation can not only alleviate pain but also uncover the specifics of the stone's characteristics, guiding appropriate management strategies.

- **Blood in the Urine: Visible or Detected Hematuria**

The presence of blood in the urine, whether visible or detected through laboratory tests, should prompt immediate medical attention. Hematuria is a key indicator of kidney stones and may also signal potential complications, such as urinary tract infections. Seeking medical advice promptly allows for a thorough assessment, accurate diagnosis, and the initiation of appropriate treatment.

- **Changes in Urinary Patterns: Alarming Deviations**

Significant changes in urinary patterns, including increased frequency, urgency, or difficulty in urination, warrant medical attention. These alterations may indicate the presence of kidney stones affecting the normal functioning of the urinary system. Addressing these deviations promptly allows for a comprehensive evaluation of renal health and the implementation of measures to manage and prevent further complications.

- **Nausea and Vomiting: Gastrointestinal Distress**

Persistent nausea and vomiting, particularly when accompanied by other renal symptoms, signal the need for medical evaluation. Kidney stones can induce gastrointestinal distress, and prolonged symptoms may suggest complications requiring intervention. Seeking medical attention promptly enables healthcare professionals to assess the broader impact of kidney stones on overall health.

- **Signs of Infection: Fever and Chills**

The development of fever and chills, especially in conjunction with other kidney stone symptoms, may indicate a urinary tract infection or other complications. In such cases, immediate medical attention is crucial to address the underlying infection, prevent its spread, and ensure optimal renal health.

- **Inability to Pass Urine: Potential Obstruction**

If an individual experiences an inability to pass urine, this may signify a complete blockage caused by a larger kidney stone. This constitutes a medical emergency, necessitating immediate attention to relieve the obstruction and prevent damage to the kidneys.

- **Presence of Pre-existing Medical Conditions: Tailored Care**

Individuals with pre-existing medical conditions, such as diabetes or a history of kidney disease, should be especially vigilant. Kidney stones can pose additional risks in these cases, and seeking medical attention at the onset of symptoms allows for personalized care that considers the individual's overall health context.

In the realm of kidney stones, recognizing the signs that necessitate medical attention is a proactive step toward optimal renal health. Whether prompted by pain, changes in urine, or systemic symptoms, seeking timely medical advice empowers individuals to address kidney stones effectively, mitigating discomfort and preventing potential complications.

40

CHAPTER 5: DIAGNOSTIC PROCEDURES

In the quest to unravel the mysteries of kidney stones and pave the way for effective management, accurate diagnosis is the cornerstone. This chapter explores the array of diagnostic procedures available, each serving as a unique lens through which healthcare professionals can peer into the intricacies of renal health. From non-invasive imaging techniques to laboratory analyses, these procedures play a pivotal role in deciphering the composition, size, and location of kidney stones.

Imaging Modalities: Peering into the Renal Landscape

Ultrasound Imaging:

Utilizing sound waves to create detailed images, ultrasound is a non-invasive and widely accessible diagnostic tool for kidney stones. It provides real-time visualization of the kidneys and helps identify the presence, size, and location of stones.

CT Scan (Computed Tomography):

CT scans offer a detailed and three-dimensional view of the urinary tract, enabling precise identification and characterization of kidney stones. While highly effective, the use of CT scans is often reserved for cases where ultrasound results are inconclusive or additional information is needed.

X-ray:

Traditional X-rays can capture images of kidney stones, particularly those composed of calcium. However, their effectiveness may be limited in identifying stones with different compositions, such as uric acid stones.

Laboratory Tests: Deciphering the Composition

Urinalysis:

Analysis of urine can provide valuable insights into the composition of kidney stones. Identifying elevated levels of minerals, crystals, or blood in the urine assists in pinpointing the type of stones and guiding appropriate preventive measures.

Blood Tests:

Blood tests, including serum creatinine and blood urea nitrogen (BUN), help assess kidney function and detect any impairment caused by the presence of kidney stones or associated complications.

Intravenous Pyelogram (IVP): Illuminating the Urinary Tract

IVP Imaging:

Intravenous pyelogram involves injecting a contrast dye into a vein, which then travels through the urinary tract. X-rays are taken to capture the dye's path, providing a dynamic view of the kidneys, ureters, and bladder. IVP can effectively highlight the presence and location of kidney stones.

Stone Analysis: Unraveling the Chemical Composition

Stone Retrieval and Analysis:

In cases where a stone has been passed or removed, laboratory analysis can determine its chemical composition. This information is invaluable for tailoring treatment plans and implementing targeted preventive measures.

24-Hour Urine Collection: Understanding Metabolic Factors

Metabolic Stone Evaluation:

A comprehensive assessment of urinary components over a 24-hour period can reveal metabolic factors contributing to stone formation. This includes measurements of calcium, oxalate, citrate, and other elements, guiding healthcare professionals in formulating personalized prevention strategies.

By navigating the array of diagnostic procedures available, healthcare professionals can unravel the specifics of kidney stone composition, size, and location. This wealth of information not only aids in accurate diagnosis but also forms the bedrock for crafting personalized treatment plans and preventive measures, fostering resilience in the face of renal challenges.

Imaging Techniques for Stone Diagnosis

In the intricate realm of renal health, imaging techniques serve as invaluable tools for diagnosing kidney stones. These non-invasive and advanced technologies offer healthcare professionals a window into the intricate architecture of the urinary tract, helping identify the presence, composition, size, and location of kidney stones. This section explores the key imaging modalities employed in the diagnostic journey of kidney stones.

Ultrasound Imaging: Visualizing in Real-Time

- **Principle:**
Ultrasound imaging utilizes high-frequency sound waves to create detailed images of the kidneys and urinary tract. It is non-invasive and provides real-time

visualization, making it an accessible and widely employed diagnostic tool.

- **Application:**

Identification of Stones: Ultrasound is effective in identifying the presence of kidney stones, offering insights into their size, location, and impact on the urinary tract.

Dynamic Observation: The real-time nature of ultrasound allows for dynamic observation, capturing the movement and behavior of stones during the examination.

- **Advantages:**

Non-invasiveness: Ultrasound is a non-invasive procedure, making it safe and suitable for various patient populations.

Real-time Imaging: The ability to observe the kidneys in real-time enhances the diagnostic capabilities of ultrasound.

CT Scan (Computed Tomography): Three-Dimensional Precision

- **Principle:**

Computed Tomography (CT) scans involve the use of X-rays to create detailed, cross-sectional images of the urinary tract. These images are reconstructed into a three-dimensional representation, providing precise insights into the anatomy.

- **Application:**

Detailed Visualization: CT scans offer a comprehensive and detailed view of the urinary tract, aiding in the identification of stones and assessing their size, composition, and location.

Distinguishing Stone Types: CT scans are particularly effective in differentiating between various types of kidney stones.

- **Advantages:**

High Precision: CT scans provide high-resolution images, allowing for accurate diagnosis and characterization of kidney stones.

Quick and Comprehensive: CT scans are efficient, providing a quick yet comprehensive assessment of renal anatomy.

X-ray: Capturing Calcium-Based Stones

- **Principle:**

Traditional X-rays use ionizing radiation to capture images of the urinary tract. X-rays are effective in identifying calcium-based stones.

- **Application:**

Identification of Calcium Stones: X-rays are particularly effective in capturing images of kidney stones composed of calcium.

Quick Evaluation: X-rays offer a rapid evaluation, making them useful in emergent situations.

- **Advantages:**

Widely Available: X-rays are a readily available and cost-effective imaging modality.

Calcium Stone Identification: X-rays are particularly adept at identifying and characterizing calcium-based stones.

These imaging techniques, each with its unique strengths, play a pivotal role in the diagnostic journey of kidney stones. The choice of modality often depends on factors such as the clinical context, urgency of diagnosis, and specific characteristics of the stones. By harnessing the capabilities of ultrasound, CT scans, and X-rays, healthcare professionals can decipher the renal landscape with precision, guiding tailored treatment plans and preventive strategies for individuals grappling with kidney stones.

Laboratory Tests and Analysis

Beyond the realm of imaging, laboratory tests stand as crucial pillars in the diagnostic arsenal for kidney stones. These tests offer insights into the composition of urine and blood, unraveling the chemical clues that aid in characterizing the nature of the stones and assessing their impact on renal function. This section delves into the key laboratory tests employed in the diagnosis of kidney stones.

Urinalysis: Unveiling Urinary Clues

- **Purpose:**

Detecting Blood in Urine (Hematuria): Urinalysis is instrumental in identifying the presence of blood in the urine, a common indicator of kidney stones.

Assessing Mineral Levels: It helps assess the levels of minerals, crystals, and other substances in the urine, offering clues about the composition of kidney stones.

- **Application:**

Identifying Stone Types: Elevated levels of specific minerals in urinalysis provide valuable information for identifying the type of kidney stones.

Monitoring Treatment: Urinalysis is employed to monitor the effectiveness of treatments and preventive measures.

Blood Tests: Assessing Renal Function

- **Purpose:**

Evaluating Kidney Function: Blood tests, including serum creatinine and blood urea nitrogen (BUN), assess kidney function and detect any impairment caused by kidney stones or associated complications.

- **Application:**

Renal Health Assessment: Blood tests provide an overall assessment of renal health, helping healthcare professionals gauge the impact of kidney stones on kidney function.

Guiding Treatment: Abnormalities in blood test results may guide treatment decisions and interventions.

Stone Analysis: Decoding the Composition

- **Purpose:**

Identifying Chemical Composition: When stones are passed or removed, laboratory analysis determines their chemical composition.

Guiding Treatment Plans: This information is crucial for tailoring treatment plans and preventive measures based on the specific characteristics of the stones.

- **Application:**

Personalized Prevention: Stone analysis enables personalized preventive strategies, considering the unique composition of the stones.

Informing Dietary Changes: Knowledge of stone composition guides dietary recommendations to minimize the risk of recurrence.

24-Hour Urine Collection: A Comprehensive Metabolic Snapshot

- **Purpose:**

Evaluating Metabolic Factors: This test involves collecting urine over a 24-hour period to assess levels of calcium, oxalate, citrate, and other elements, providing insights into metabolic factors contributing to stone formation.

- **Application:**

Personalized Prevention: The results of a 24-hour urine collection guide the formulation of personalized prevention strategies, addressing underlying metabolic imbalances.

Monitoring Treatment Efficacy: Periodic 24-hour urine collections help monitor the effectiveness of interventions and preventive measures.

These laboratory tests serve as invaluable tools for healthcare professionals in deciphering the renal code written by kidney stones. By analyzing urine and blood components, clinicians gain a comprehensive understanding of the composition, impact, and metabolic factors influencing stone formation. This knowledge not only aids in accurate diagnosis but forms the foundation for personalized treatment plans and preventive strategies, fostering renal resilience in the face of kidney stones.

CHAPTER 6: TYPES OF KIDNEY STONE TREATMENTS

As we embark on the journey to conquer kidney stones, a diverse array of treatment options unfolds before us. This chapter explores the multifaceted landscape of interventions designed to alleviate symptoms, facilitate stone passage, and prevent recurrence. From lifestyle modifications to medical management and surgical procedures, understanding the spectrum of treatments empowers individuals to navigate the path toward renal resilience.

Conservative Management: Letting Nature Take Its Course

Hydration: Adequate fluid intake stands as a cornerstone in the management of kidney stones. Diluting urine helps prevent the concentration of minerals that contribute to stone formation.

Pain Management: Over-the-counter pain medications, such as nonsteroidal anti-inflammatory drugs (NSAIDs), may be recommended to alleviate pain during the passage of kidney stones.

Observation and Monitoring: In cases of small stones that are likely to pass on their own, healthcare professionals may opt for a conservative approach, closely monitoring symptoms while providing supportive care.

Lifestyle Modifications: Fortifying Renal Resilience

Dietary Changes: Tailoring dietary choices to minimize the intake of substances that contribute to stone formation, such as oxalate-rich foods or foods high in purines, can be instrumental.

Calcium and Oxalate Management: Achieving a balance in calcium intake and managing oxalate-rich foods helps mitigate the risk of calcium oxalate stone formation.

Hydration Practices: Adopting habits that promote optimal hydration, such as regular water intake and avoidance of dehydration, plays a pivotal role in preventing stone recurrence.

Medications: Targeting Stone Formation Factors

Thiazide Diuretics: These medications may be prescribed to reduce the excretion of calcium in the urine, thereby lowering the risk of calcium-based stone formation.

Allopurinol: In cases where uric acid stones are prevalent, allopurinol may be prescribed to manage elevated uric acid levels and prevent stone recurrence.

Phosphate Binders: Phosphate binders help manage high levels of phosphate in the urine, a factor associated with certain types of kidney stones.

Extracorporeal Shock Wave Lithotripsy (ESWL): Breaking Stones from Afar

Principle: ESWL employs shock waves generated outside the body to break kidney stones into smaller fragments, facilitating their passage through the urinary tract.

Application: This non-invasive procedure is often employed for small to medium-sized stones, allowing for stone fragmentation without the need for surgical intervention.

Ureteroscopy: Navigating the Ureter with Precision

Principle: Ureteroscopy involves the insertion of a thin, flexible tube equipped with a camera through the urethra and bladder to directly visualize and remove stones from the urinary tract.

Application: Ureteroscopy is effective for stones located in the ureter or kidney, providing a direct and precise means of intervention.

Percutaneous Nephrolithotomy (PCNL): Surgical Precision

Principle: PCNL is a surgical procedure where a small incision is made, and a tube is inserted directly into the kidney to remove or break down large or complex stones.

Application: PCNL is often reserved for larger stones or those that cannot be effectively treated with less invasive methods.

Metabolic Evaluation and Follow-Up: A Comprehensive Approach

Metabolic Stone Evaluation: Periodic assessments of metabolic factors, including 24-hour urine collections, guide ongoing preventive strategies and treatment adjustments.

Regular Follow-Up: Long-term management involves regular follow-up appointments to monitor kidney health, assess the effectiveness of interventions, and tailor strategies to prevent stone recurrence.

By navigating the diverse landscape of kidney stone treatments, individuals can work in tandem with healthcare professionals to tailor approaches that align with their unique circumstances. Whether through conservative measures, lifestyle modifications, medications, or surgical interventions, the goal remains steadfast: to conquer kidney stones and foster renal resilience on the path to sustained well-being.

Medical Management

In the intricate tapestry of kidney stone management, medical interventions play a pivotal role, offering precision in addressing specific factors that contribute to stone formation. This section explores the diverse array of pharmaceutical strategies employed to mitigate symptoms, alter urinary chemistry, and prevent the recurrence of kidney stones.

Thiazide Diuretics: Regulating Calcium in the Urine

- **Mechanism:**

Thiazide diuretics, such as hydrochlorothiazide, function by promoting the reabsorption of calcium in the kidneys, reducing its excretion in the urine. This can be particularly beneficial for individuals prone to calcium-based stone formation.

- **Application:**

Reducing Calcium Excretion: Thiazides help lower the levels of calcium in the urine, addressing a key factor in the development of calcium oxalate stones.

Preventing Recurrence: Prescribed as part of a comprehensive treatment plan, thiazides contribute to the prevention of recurrent kidney stones.

Allopurinol: Managing Uric Acid Levels

- **Mechanism:**

Allopurinol is a medication that inhibits the production of uric acid in the body, thereby lowering uric acid levels in the urine. This is particularly relevant for individuals susceptible to uric acid stone formation.

- **Application:**

Uric Acid Stone Prevention: By reducing uric acid levels, allopurinol helps prevent the formation of uric acid stones.

Long-Term Management: Allopurinol may be prescribed as a long-term measure to maintain optimal uric acid levels and minimize stone recurrence.

Potassium Citrate: Alkalizing the Urine

- **Mechanism:**

Potassium citrate works by increasing the urinary pH, making the urine less acidic. This can help prevent the formation of certain types of stones, such as uric acid and cystine stones.

- **Application:**

Urinary Alkalization: Potassium citrate helps create an environment in the urinary tract that is less conducive to the formation of acidic stones.

Cystine Stone Prevention: In cases of cystine stones, which form in acidic urine, potassium citrate can be particularly effective.

Phosphate Binders: Managing Phosphate Levels

- **Mechanism:**

Phosphate binders, such as calcium-based antacids, help limit the absorption of phosphate in the digestive tract. This can be relevant in managing phosphate levels in individuals prone to certain types of kidney stones.

- **Application:**

Reducing Phosphate in Urine: Phosphate binders contribute to lowering phosphate levels in the urine, addressing a factor associated with stone formation.

Preventing Calcium Phosphate Stones: In individuals susceptible to calcium phosphate stones, phosphate binders can play a preventive role.

Antibiotics: Addressing Infection-Related Stones

- **Mechanism:**

Antibiotics may be prescribed to treat or prevent urinary tract infections (UTIs), which can contribute to the formation of struvite stones.

- **Application:**

Infection Management: Antibiotics help treat bacterial infections that may lead to the formation of struvite stones.

Preventing Recurrence: In cases where recurrent UTIs contribute to stone formation, long-term antibiotic prophylaxis may be considered.

Individualized Approaches: Tailoring Medications to Stone Composition

Stone Analysis Guidance: The results of stone analysis, which identifies the specific composition of kidney stones, guide the selection of medications tailored to the individual's stone type.

Personalized Prevention: By understanding the unique characteristics of the stones, healthcare professionals can customize pharmaceutical interventions to target the underlying factors contributing to stone formation.

In the realm of medical management for kidney stones, precision is key. By leveraging pharmaceutical interventions that specifically address the components of stone formation, healthcare professionals can provide targeted strategies to alleviate symptoms, prevent recurrence, and promote renal resilience. These medications, often integrated into a comprehensive treatment plan, empower individuals on the path to conquering kidney stones and sustaining optimal renal health.

Surgical Interventions

When kidney stones present formidable challenges that transcend non-invasive measures, surgical interventions emerge as powerful tools in the quest for renal resilience. This section explores the diverse array of surgical procedures designed to address large, complex, or stubborn stones, offering precision and efficacy in the face of significant renal obstacles.

Extracorporeal Shock Wave Lithotripsy (ESWL): Breaking Stones from Afar

- **Principle:**
ESWL employs shock waves generated outside the body to break kidney stones into smaller fragments, facilitating their passage through the urinary tract.

- **Application:**

Non-Invasive Stone Fragmentation: ESWL is particularly effective for small to medium-sized stones that can be shattered without the need for surgical incisions.

Wide Applicability: This non-invasive approach is suitable for various types of stones and is often employed as an outpatient procedure.

Ureteroscopy: Precision Navigation of the Ureter

- **Principle:**

Ureteroscopy involves the insertion of a thin, flexible tube equipped with a camera through the urethra and bladder to directly visualize and remove stones from the urinary tract.

- **Application:**

Direct Stone Removal: Ureteroscopy allows for the precise visualization and removal of stones located in the ureter or kidney.

Minimally Invasive: With advancements in technology, ureteroscopy has become a minimally invasive approach, often performed as an outpatient procedure.

Percutaneous Nephrolithotomy (PCNL): Surgical Precision

- **Principle:**

PCNL is a surgical procedure where a small incision is made, and a tube is inserted directly into the kidney to remove or break down large or complex stones.

- **Application:**

Large Stone Management: PCNL is particularly effective for larger stones or those that cannot be effectively treated with less invasive methods.

Comprehensive Stone Clearance: This surgical intervention allows for a comprehensive approach to stone removal, often achieving complete clearance in a single session.

Laser Lithotripsy: Precision Stone Disintegration

- **Principle:**

Laser lithotripsy involves the use of laser energy to break down kidney stones into smaller fragments, facilitating their removal.

- **Application:**

Targeted Stone Disintegration: Laser lithotripsy provides a precise and targeted approach to breaking down stones, often used in conjunction with other procedures like ureteroscopy.

Effective for Various Stone Types: This method is effective for a range of stone compositions, offering versatility in stone management.

Open Surgery: Reserved for Complex Cases

- **Principle:**

In rare and complex cases, open surgery may be considered, involving a larger incision for direct access to the kidneys or urinary tract.

- **Application:**

Complex Stone Scenarios: Open surgery is reserved for situations where other interventions are not feasible or effective, such as extremely large stones or anatomical challenges.

Multidisciplinary Approach: In such cases, a multidisciplinary team collaborates to ensure the success of the surgical procedure.

Robotic-Assisted Surgery: Advancements in Precision

- **Principle:**

Robotic-assisted surgery involves the use of robotic systems to enhance the precision and maneuverability of surgical instruments during procedures like ureteroscopy or pyelolithotomy.

- **Application:**

Enhanced Precision: Robotic-assisted surgery allows for enhanced precision, making it particularly useful in intricate procedures involving stone removal.

Minimally Invasive Approach: While still considered minimally invasive, robotic-assisted surgery provides improved control and dexterity for the surgeon.

In the realm of surgical interventions for kidney stones, each method is carefully selected based on the specific characteristics of the stones, the patient's health, and the complexities of the case. From non-invasive approaches like ESWL to more intricate procedures such as PCNL or robotic-assisted surgery, these interventions stand as powerful allies in the pursuit of conquering kidney stones and restoring optimal renal health.

CHAPTER 7: PAIN MANAGEMENT

As individuals navigate the tumultuous waters of kidney stone challenges, the surges of pain can be both intense and unpredictable. This chapter explores the nuances of pain management, shedding light on strategies to alleviate discomfort, enhance resilience, and empower individuals on their journey to conquer kidney stones.

Nonsteroidal Anti-Inflammatory Drugs (NSAIDs): Easing the Renal Symphony

- **Mechanism:**
NSAIDs, such as ibuprofen or naproxen, are commonly employed to alleviate pain and reduce inflammation associated with kidney stones.

- **Application:**
Pain Relief: NSAIDs are effective in providing pain relief, particularly when renal pain is caused by inflammation or muscle spasms.

71

Anti-Inflammatory Action: By mitigating inflammation, NSAIDs contribute to the overall reduction of discomfort associated with kidney stones.

Acetaminophen: A Gentle Analgesic Approach

- **Mechanism:**

Acetaminophen is an analgesic with pain-relieving properties, but it lacks the anti-inflammatory effects of NSAIDs.

- **Application:**

Pain Management: Acetaminophen is a suitable option for pain management when inflammation is not a predominant factor in renal discomfort.

Liver Considerations: It is particularly considered for individuals who may need to avoid NSAIDs due to liver concerns.

Opioid Analgesics: Addressing Severe Pain

- **Mechanism:**

Opioid analgesics, such as oxycodone or morphine, are potent pain relievers that act on the central nervous system.

- **Application:**

Severe Pain Relief: Opioids are reserved for cases of severe pain that may not be adequately controlled by NSAIDs or acetaminophen.

Short-Term Use: Due to the potential for dependence and side effects, opioids are typically prescribed for short-term use.

Alpha-Blockers: Facilitating Stone Passage

- **Mechanism:**

Alpha-blockers, like tamsulosin, relax the muscles in the ureter, facilitating the passage of kidney stones.

- **Application:**

Assisting Stone Passage: Alpha-blockers may be prescribed to help ease the passage of stones through the ureter, reducing pain and discomfort.

Improved Urinary Flow: These medications can enhance urinary flow, aiding in the expulsion of stones.

Intravenous (IV) Pain Medications: Rapid Relief in Emergency Settings

- **Mechanism:**

In emergency settings or severe cases, healthcare professionals may administer pain medications intravenously for rapid relief.

- **Application:**

Immediate Relief: IV pain medications provide swift relief for individuals experiencing acute and severe renal pain.

Hospital Settings: Administration is typically done in a hospital or emergency setting under close medical supervision.

Localized Heat Therapy: Soothing the Renal Landscape

- **Mechanism:**

Applying heat to the affected area, such as using a heating pad or warm compress, can help relax muscles and alleviate pain.

- **Application:**

Muscle Relaxation: Heat therapy promotes muscle relaxation, potentially easing the muscle spasms associated with kidney stone pain.

Complementary Approach: Used in conjunction with medications, heat therapy offers a complementary and comforting dimension to pain management.

Fluid Intake: Hydration as a Natural Analgesic

- **Mechanism:**

Adequate fluid intake helps dilute urine, reducing the concentration of minerals that contribute to stone formation.

- **Application:**

Natural Analgesic: Hydration serves as a natural analgesic by promoting the passage of stones and minimizing their impact on the urinary tract.

Preventive Measure: Ongoing hydration is a crucial preventive measure, reducing the risk of stone recurrence.

Behavioral and Relaxation Techniques: Calming the Waters

- **Mechanism:**

Techniques such as deep breathing, guided imagery, or meditation can help individuals manage stress and cope with pain.

- **Application:**

Stress Reduction: Behavioral and relaxation techniques contribute to stress reduction, potentially easing the emotional and physical toll of kidney stone pain.

Comprehensive Pain Management: When integrated into a comprehensive pain management plan, these techniques enhance overall well-being.

By navigating the spectrum of pain management strategies, individuals facing the challenges of kidney stones can find tailored approaches that align with their unique needs. From pharmaceutical interventions to complementary techniques, the goal is not only to alleviate discomfort but to empower individuals on their journey to conquer kidney stones and foster resilience in the face of renal challenges.

Coping with Kidney Stone Pain

Facing the waves of pain that accompany kidney stones requires not only medical intervention but also effective coping strategies to navigate the challenges with resilience and fortitude. This section delves into practical and psychological approaches to cope with kidney stone pain, offering insights into managing discomfort and maintaining a positive outlook throughout the journey.

Understanding the Pain: Knowledge as Empowerment

- **Education:**

- Understanding the nature of kidney stone pain, its causes, and the potential fluctuations in intensity can empower individuals to face the challenges with a sense of knowledge and preparedness.

- Seeking information from healthcare professionals and reliable sources fosters a proactive approach to pain management.

Medication Adherence: Consistency in Relief

- **Follow Healthcare Recommendations:**
- Adhering to prescribed medications as directed by healthcare professionals ensures consistent pain relief.
- Communicating any concerns or side effects promptly allows for adjustments in the pain management plan.

Hydration: The Fluid Path to Relief

- **Adequate Water Intake:**
- Maintaining proper hydration is crucial for diluting urine and promoting the passage of stones, potentially reducing pain.

- Carrying a water bottle and setting regular reminders can help establish and maintain healthy hydration habits.

Warm Compress and Baths: Soothing the Discomfort

- **Localized Heat Therapy:**
- Applying a warm compress or taking a warm bath can help relax muscles and alleviate discomfort.
- Heat therapy serves as a simple and comforting technique to complement medical interventions.

Breathing Exercises: Calming the Storm Within

- **Deep Breathing:**
- Engaging in deep breathing exercises helps manage stress and provides a sense of control during painful episodes.
- Focusing on slow, deep breaths can distract from pain and promote a sense of calm.

Distraction Techniques: Shifting Focus

- **Engaging Hobbies or Activities:**

- Immerse yourself in activities or hobbies that capture your attention and divert focus from pain.

- Watching movies, reading, or listening to music can be effective distraction techniques.

Emotional Support: Building a Solid Shoreline

- **Family and Friends:**

- Seeking support from family and friends can provide emotional reassurance and understanding.

- Sharing experiences with loved ones fosters a sense of connectedness and reduces feelings of isolation.

Mindfulness and Meditation: Embracing the Present Moment

- **Mindfulness Practices:**

- Mindfulness and meditation techniques promote an awareness of the present moment, helping individuals manage pain and stress.

- Guided imagery or meditation apps can be valuable tools in cultivating a mindful mindset.

Communicating with Healthcare Professionals: Partners in Pain Management

- **Open Communication:**
  - Establishing open communication with healthcare professionals is essential for addressing concerns, adjusting pain management plans, and ensuring personalized care.
  - Regular check-ins allow for ongoing evaluation of pain management strategies.

Mental Health Support: Nurturing Emotional Well-Being

- **Therapeutic Support:**
  - Seeking the guidance of mental health professionals can be instrumental in managing the emotional toll of chronic pain.

- Therapists can provide coping strategies, stress management techniques, and a supportive space to navigate the psychological impact of kidney stone pain.

Coping with kidney stone pain is a multifaceted journey that encompasses not only medical interventions but also psychological and lifestyle strategies. By adopting a holistic approach to pain management, individuals can cultivate resilience, minimize the impact of discomfort, and navigate the challenges with a sense of empowerment and well-being.

Medications and Home Remedies

As individuals encounter the challenges posed by kidney stones, a combination of medications and home remedies serves as a dynamic toolkit for managing symptoms, promoting stone passage, and preventing recurrence. This section explores the diverse array of pharmaceutical interventions and practical strategies that individuals can incorporate into their daily lives to foster renal resilience.

Nonsteroidal Anti-Inflammatory Drugs (NSAIDs): Tackling Inflammation and Pain

- **Mechanism:**

- NSAIDs, such as ibuprofen or naproxen, target inflammation and alleviate pain associated with kidney stones.

- **Application:**

Pain Relief: NSAIDs are effective in managing the discomfort caused by inflammation, making them valuable for individuals experiencing renal pain.

Anti-Inflammatory Action: By mitigating inflammation, NSAIDs contribute to reducing the overall impact of kidney stone-related pain.

Alpha-Blockers: Facilitating Stone Passage

- **Mechanism:**

Alpha-blockers, like tamsulosin, relax the muscles in the ureter, facilitating the passage of kidney stones.

- **Application:**

Assisting Stone Passage: Alpha-blockers may be prescribed to help stones move more easily through the urinary tract, reducing pain and expediting stone expulsion.

Pain Management Medications: Tailoring Relief

- **Medication Choices:**

Acetaminophen, opioids, or other pain management medications may be prescribed based on the severity of pain.

- **Application:**

Short-Term Relief: Pain management medications are often used for short durations to provide immediate relief during acute episodes of kidney stone pain.

Hydration Practices: The Natural Elixir for Stone Passage

- **Adequate Water Intake:**

Ensuring sufficient daily water intake helps dilute urine, reducing the concentration of minerals that contribute to stone formation.

- **Application:**

Promoting Stone Passage: Hydration is a natural strategy to facilitate the passage of stones, potentially minimizing pain and discomfort.

Preventive Measure: Maintaining consistent hydration is a preventive measure against stone recurrence.

Dietary Modifications: Crafting a Kidney-Friendly Plate

- **Calcium and Oxalate Management:**

Adjusting dietary choices to balance calcium and oxalate intake helps prevent the formation of certain types of kidney stones.

Application:

- **Tailored Nutrition**: Dietary modifications, such as reducing oxalate-rich foods or adjusting calcium intake, contribute to stone prevention and overall renal health.

Lemonade Therapy: Harnessing the Power of Citrate

- **Mechanism:**

Drinking lemonade, particularly with added citric acid, can increase urinary citrate levels, which inhibits stone formation.

- **Application:**

Citrate Boost: Lemonade therapy is a home remedy that provides a natural source of citric acid, potentially reducing the risk of certain types of kidney stones.

Dietary Fiber: Supporting Overall Digestive Health

- **Mechanism:**

Adequate dietary fiber intake supports digestive health and may help regulate calcium and oxalate absorption.

- **Application:**

Balanced Digestion: A diet rich in fiber promotes overall digestive health, potentially contributing to optimal nutrient absorption and stone prevention.

Herbal Remedies: Exploring Natural Options

- **Mechanism:**

Some individuals explore herbal remedies, such as herbal teas or supplements, which are believed to have potential benefits for kidney stone management.

- **Application:**

Caution Advised: While herbal remedies may be considered, it's essential to exercise caution and consult healthcare professionals due to potential interactions with medications.

Physical Activity: Promoting General Well-Being

- **Mechanism:**

Regular physical activity supports overall well-being, potentially reducing stress and promoting optimal metabolic function.

- **Application:**

Stress Reduction: Exercise contributes to stress reduction, which can be beneficial for individuals managing the emotional toll of kidney stone challenges.

Stress Management Techniques: Nurturing Emotional Resilience

- **Mindfulness and Relaxation:**

Engaging in mindfulness practices, relaxation techniques, or activities that promote emotional well-being can contribute to resilience in the face of kidney stone challenges.

- **Application:**

Holistic Well-Being: Stress management techniques complement medical interventions, fostering a holistic approach to kidney stone management.

In the realm of kidney stone management, the integration of medications and home remedies forms a comprehensive strategy for alleviating symptoms, promoting stone passage, and preventing recurrence. By adopting a tailored approach that aligns with individual preferences and health needs, individuals can navigate the path to relief and foster resilience in the face of renal challenges.

CHAPTER 8: DIETARY STRATEGIES FOR PREVENTION

In the pursuit of kidney stone prevention, dietary strategies play a central role, offering a proactive and personalized approach to mitigating the risk of stone formation. This chapter delves into the intricacies of dietary choices, providing insights into nutrition, hydration, and lifestyle adjustments that empower individuals to foster renal resilience and reduce the likelihood of kidney stones.

Hydration: The Foundation of Prevention

- **Adequate Water Intake:**
 - Maintaining optimal hydration is paramount for preventing kidney stones.
 - Adequate water dilutes urine, reducing the concentration of minerals that can lead to stone formation.

- **Application:**

Water as a Habit: Cultivate a habit of regular water intake throughout the day, aiming for at least 8 glasses (64 ounces) or more, depending on individual needs. **Urine Color as a Guide**: Monitor urine color; a pale yellow hue indicates proper hydration.

Calcium Balance: The Crucial Equation

- **Calcium-Rich Foods:**

 - Include sources of dietary calcium in your meals, such as dairy products, leafy greens, and fortified foods.
 - Balanced calcium intake is essential for preventing oxalate absorption and the formation of calcium oxalate stones.

- **Application:**

Optimal Serving Sizes: Choose appropriate serving sizes of calcium-rich foods to maintain a balance without excess.

Supplements with Caution: If using calcium supplements, consult healthcare professionals to ensure they align with individual needs.

Sodium Moderation: A Salty Symphony

- **Reduced Sodium Intake:**

- Limit the consumption of high-sodium foods, such as processed foods, canned soups, and salty snacks.

- High sodium can lead to increased calcium excretion in the urine, contributing to stone formation.

- **Application:**

Read Food Labels: Be vigilant in reading food labels to identify and reduce high-sodium choices.

Cooking at Home: Preparing meals at home allows for better control over salt content.

Oxalate Awareness: Balancing Oxalate-Rich Foods

- **Moderation of Oxalate Intake:**

- Be mindful of foods high in oxalates, such as spinach, beets, nuts, and chocolate.

- While oxalates are a factor in some kidney stones, a balanced approach is key.

- **Application:**

Variety in the Diet: Incorporate a diverse range of foods to avoid excessive intake of any single high-oxalate item.

Cooking Techniques: Certain cooking methods, like boiling, can reduce oxalate content in vegetables.

Phosphorus Control: Balancing Mineral Harmony

- **Phosphorus-Rich Foods:**

  - Limit consumption of phosphorus-rich foods, such as colas, red meats, and processed foods.

  - High phosphorus levels can contribute to the formation of calcium phosphate stones.

- **Application:**

Diversify Protein Sources: Opt for a mix of protein sources, including lean meats, poultry, fish, and plant-based options.

Phosphorus Content Awareness: Be aware of the phosphorus content in food choices and make informed decisions.

Limiting Animal Proteins: Striking a Protein Balance

- **Moderation in Animal Proteins:**

  - Limit intake of red meats, organ meats, and high-purine animal products.
  - Excessive animal protein consumption can increase uric acid levels, contributing to stone formation.

- **Application:**

  Vegetarian Alternatives: Explore plant-based protein sources, including legumes, tofu, and nuts.
  Balanced Protein Intake: Achieve a balanced protein intake that aligns with individual nutritional needs.

Citrus Fruits and Beverages: Citrate for Stone Prevention

- **Incorporating Citrus Fruits:**

  - Include citrus fruits like lemons, oranges, and limes in your diet.
  - Citrate from citrus fruits inhibits stone formation by binding with calcium in the urine.

- **Application:**

Citrus-Infused Water: Create refreshing beverages by infusing water with citrus slices.

Citrus as Snacks: Snack on citrus fruits or add them to salads for a flavorful and kidney-friendly twist.

Balanced Diet and Weight Management: Holistic Wellness Approach

- **Nutrient-Rich Diet:**

- Embrace a diet rich in fruits, vegetables, whole grains, and lean proteins.

- A balanced diet promotes overall health and reduces the risk factors associated with kidney stone formation.

- **Application:**

Portion Control: Practice portion control to maintain a healthy weight.

Regular Physical Activity: Incorporate regular exercise to support weight management and overall well-being.

Limiting Sugar and High-Fructose Corn Syrup: Sweetening Wisely

- **Reducing Added Sugars:**

- Minimize the consumption of sugary beverages and foods with high-fructose corn syrup.

- Elevated fructose levels can contribute to the formation of uric acid stones.

- **Application:**

Natural Sweeteners: Opt for natural sweeteners like honey or maple syrup in moderation.

Reading Labels: Check food labels for added sugars and choose alternatives with lower sugar content.

Regular Monitoring and Adjustments: Personalized Prevention Journey

- **Periodic Stone Analysis:**

Periodic stone analysis, guided by healthcare professionals, helps tailor dietary strategies based on stone composition.

Application:

Consulting Healthcare Professionals: Regular consultations with healthcare professionals allow for adjustments to dietary strategies based on individual health needs.

Tracking Dietary Changes: Maintain a food diary to track dietary changes and identify patterns related to kidney stone risk.

By embracing these dietary strategies, individuals can proactively engage in kidney stone prevention, fostering renal resilience and overall well-being. These principles, when tailored to individual needs and accompanied by regular healthcare consultations, empower individuals on a personalized journey to conquer kidney stone challenges through the nourishing embrace of dietary wisdom.

Hydration and Its Role

In the intricate dance of bodily functions, few partners are as essential as water. Hydration emerges as a cornerstone in the prevention of kidney stones, playing a pivotal role in maintaining urinary health, diluting mineral concentrations, and fostering an environment that discourages the formation of these crystalline structures within the kidneys. This section delves into the significance of hydration and its multifaceted impact on renal well-being.

Dilution of Urine: Water as the Elixir of Balance

- **Mineral Concentration Control:**

- Adequate hydration ensures that urine is appropriately diluted, preventing the accumulation of minerals like calcium and oxalate that can contribute to stone formation.

- Diluted urine reduces the likelihood of mineral crystals clumping together and forming the solid core of kidney stones.

- **Application:**

Clear or Light Yellow Urine: The color of urine is a visible indicator of hydration levels. A pale yellow or clear appearance suggests proper hydration, while dark yellow or concentrated urine may indicate dehydration.

Regular Water Intake: Establish a habit of regular water intake throughout the day, aiming to maintain optimal hydration.

Stone Prevention for Various Types: A Unified Approach

- **Calcium Oxalate Stones:**

For individuals prone to calcium oxalate stones, adequate hydration helps prevent the crystallization of calcium and oxalate, reducing the risk of stone formation.

- **Uric Acid Stones:**

Hydration is particularly crucial for preventing uric acid stones, as it helps maintain a more alkaline urine pH, inhibiting the formation of uric acid crystals.

- **Calcium Phosphate Stones:**

In the case of calcium phosphate stones, proper hydration prevents the concentration of calcium and phosphate, minimizing the likelihood of stone development.

Stone Passage Facilitation: Easing the Journey

- **Reducing Stone Size and Agglomeration:**
- Hydration aids in the passage of small stones by reducing their size and preventing them from clumping together.
- It promotes a smoother journey through the urinary tract, potentially minimizing pain and discomfort.

- **Application:**

Pain Alleviation: Adequate hydration can alleviate pain during the passage of stones by facilitating their movement through the urinary system.

Increased Urinary Flow: The enhanced flow of urine helps flush out small stones, preventing their aggregation and promoting a more comfortable passage.

Optimal Hydration Practices: Beyond Quantity Alone

- **Individualized Water Needs:**

- The optimal amount of water varies among individuals based on factors such as age, weight, activity level, and climate.

- Healthcare professionals can provide personalized guidance on water intake tailored to individual needs.

- **Application:**

Water-Rich Foods: Incorporate water-rich foods, such as fruits and vegetables, into the diet to complement fluid intake.

Hydration Awareness: Stay mindful of hydration needs, especially during physical activity, hot weather, or illness, when fluid requirements may increase.

Prevention of Recurrent Stones: A Long-Term Commitment

- **Chronic Kidney Stone Prevention:**

- Hydration is a cornerstone in the long-term management and prevention of recurrent kidney stones.

- Regular and sustained hydration contributes to an ongoing reduction in the risk of stone formation.

- **Application:**

Establishing Hydration Habits: Cultivate habits that promote consistent hydration, making it an integral part of daily life.

Healthcare Professional Guidance: Individuals with a history of kidney stones should seek guidance from healthcare professionals to tailor hydration practices to their specific needs.

Holistic Well-Being: Beyond Stone Prevention

- **Overall Renal Health:**

- Beyond stone prevention, hydration promotes overall renal health by supporting the kidneys' ability to filter waste and maintain electrolyte balance.

- Proper hydration contributes to the optimal functioning of the urinary system.

- **Application:**

Incorporating Hydration into Lifestyle: Integrate hydration into lifestyle choices, recognizing its role not only in kidney stone prevention but in fostering holistic well-being.

Educating Others: Spread awareness about the importance of hydration for kidney health, contributing to a culture of proactive renal care.

In the symphony of bodily functions, hydration emerges as a conductor, orchestrating the delicate balance necessary for kidney stone prevention. Beyond a simple act of thirst quenching, adequate hydration is a proactive investment in renal resilience, offering a natural and accessible strategy for nurturing the health of these vital organs. This section encourages a mindful embrace of hydration as a fundamental pillar in the journey toward sustained renal well-being.

Kidney Stone-Friendly Diets

Navigating the realm of kidney stone prevention involves not only understanding the types and causes of stones but also adopting dietary strategies that promote renal well-being. This section explores the principles of kidney stone-friendly diets, emphasizing the incorporation of nutrient-rich foods and mindful choices to reduce the risk of stone formation and foster resilience in the intricate landscape of renal health.

Adequate Hydration: The Cornerstone of Kidney Stone-Friendly Diets

- **Water as a Primary Beverage:**
- Prioritize water as the primary beverage in kidney stone-friendly diets.
- Adequate hydration helps prevent the concentration of minerals that contribute to stone formation.

- **Application:**
Hydration Throughout the Day: Establish a routine of regular water intake throughout the day to maintain optimal hydration.
Citrus-Infused Water: Enhance hydration with citrus-infused water, as citrus fruits provide citrate that inhibits stone formation.

Calcium-Rich Foods: Striking a Balance

- **Dietary Calcium Inclusion:**

 - Include moderate amounts of dietary calcium from sources such as low-fat dairy products, leafy greens, and fortified foods.

 - Adequate calcium intake binds with oxalates in the digestive system, reducing their absorption and lowering the risk of calcium oxalate stones.

- **Application:**

Portion Control: Consume calcium-rich foods in appropriate portion sizes to maintain a balance without excess.

Consultation with Healthcare Professionals: Seek guidance from healthcare professionals for personalized calcium recommendations based on individual health needs.

Limiting Sodium Intake: A Salty Balancing Act

- **Reduced Sodium Choices:**

 - Limit the consumption of high-sodium foods, such as processed foods, canned soups, and salty snacks.

- High sodium levels can lead to increased calcium excretion in the urine, contributing to stone formation.

- **Application:**

Cooking at Home: Prepare meals at home to have better control over salt content.

Exploring Herbs and Spices: Enhance flavor with herbs and spices as alternatives to excess salt.

Moderating Oxalate Intake: Mindful Choices

- **Balanced Oxalate Consumption:**

- Be mindful of foods high in oxalates, such as spinach, beets, nuts, and chocolate.

- While oxalates are a factor in some kidney stones, moderation and a diverse diet are key.

Application:

Variety in Diet: Incorporate a variety of foods to avoid excessive intake of any single high-oxalate item.

Cooking Techniques: Certain cooking methods, like boiling, can reduce oxalate content in vegetables.

Balanced Protein Intake: Diverse Protein Sources

- **Diversifying Protein Sources:**
- Opt for a mix of protein sources, including lean meats, poultry, fish, legumes, and plant-based options.
- Limiting high-purine animal products helps prevent the formation of uric acid stones.

- **Application:**

Vegetarian Alternatives: Explore plant-based protein sources for variety and kidney-friendly options.

Portion Moderation: Practice portion control to achieve a balanced protein intake.

Phosphorus Control: Maintaining Mineral Harmony

- **Phosphorus-Rich Foods Moderation:**
- Limit the consumption of phosphorus-rich foods, such as colas, red meats, and processed foods.
- High phosphorus levels can contribute to the formation of calcium phosphate stones.

- **Application:**

Awareness of Phosphorus Content: Be conscious of phosphorus content in food choices and make informed decisions.

Balanced Diet Planning: Plan meals for a balanced distribution of nutrients, including phosphorus.

Citrus Fruits and Beverages: A Zest for Citrate

- **Incorporating Citrus Fruits:**

 - Include citrus fruits like lemons, oranges, and limes in kidney stone-friendly diets.

 - Citrate from citrus fruits inhibits stone formation by binding with calcium in the urine.

- **Application:**

Citrus-Infused Dishes: Incorporate citrus fruits into dishes, salads, or desserts for added flavor.

Snacking on Citrus: Enjoy citrus fruits as snacks for a refreshing and kidney-friendly twist.

Fiber-Rich Foods: Supporting Digestive Harmony

- **Balanced Fiber Intake:**

- Include fiber-rich foods like fruits, vegetables, and whole grains to support digestive health.

- Adequate fiber intake may help regulate calcium and oxalate absorption.

- **Application:**

Whole Grain Choices: Opt for whole grains over refined grains for increased fiber content.

Daily Fiber Goals: Aim for recommended daily fiber intake for overall well-being.

Limiting Added Sugars: A Sweetened Approach

- **Reducing Added Sugars:**

- Minimize the consumption of sugary beverages and foods with high-fructose corn syrup.

- Elevated fructose levels can contribute to the formation of uric acid stones.

- **Application:**

Natural Sweeteners: Choose natural sweeteners like honey or maple syrup in moderation.

Reading Food Labels: Check labels for added sugars and opt for alternatives with lower sugar content.

Consultation and Customization: Personalizing Kidney Stone-Friendly Diets

- **Healthcare Professional Guidance:**

  - Consult with healthcare professionals for personalized dietary guidance, especially for individuals with a history of kidney stones.
  - Periodic evaluations allow for adjustments to kidney stone-friendly diets based on individual health needs.

Application:

Monitoring Stone Composition: Periodic stone analysis guides dietary adjustments based on stone composition.

Communication with Professionals: Maintain open communication with healthcare professionals for ongoing support and personalized advice.

Embarking on a kidney stone-friendly diet is a journey of proactive renal care, where nutrient-rich choices and mindful selections intertwine to create a symphony of well-being. Through these dietary principles, individuals can embrace a nourishing approach that not only reduces the risk of kidney stone formation but also contributes to overall renal resilience and optimal health.

CHAPTER 9: LIFESTYLE MODIFICATIONS

In the pursuit of kidney stone prevention and fostering renal resilience, lifestyle modifications serve as transformative pillars that extend beyond dietary considerations. This chapter explores a spectrum of lifestyle adjustments, encompassing physical activity, stress management, and environmental factors, to empower individuals on their journey to conquer kidney stones and cultivate lasting well-being.

Regular Physical Activity: Nurturing Whole-Body Wellness

- **Exercise for Metabolic Health:**
  - Engage in regular physical activity to support metabolic health and contribute to overall well-being.
  - Exercise promotes optimal weight management and metabolic function, reducing risk factors for kidney stone formation.

- **Application:**

Aerobic Activities: Incorporate aerobic exercises, such as brisk walking, jogging, or swimming, for cardiovascular health.

Strength Training: Include strength training exercises to enhance muscle tone and support overall metabolic function.

Weight Management: Striking a Balance for Renal Health

- **Maintaining a Healthy Weight:**

 - Achieve and maintain a healthy weight to reduce the risk of kidney stone formation.

 - Excess body weight is associated with metabolic changes that can contribute to stone development.

- **Application:**

Balanced Nutrition: Combine a kidney stone-friendly diet with portion control to support weight management.

Consultation with Healthcare Professionals: Seek guidance from healthcare professionals for personalized weight management strategies.

Stress Reduction Techniques: Soothing the Renal Landscape

- **Mindfulness and Relaxation:**
  - Incorporate stress reduction techniques, such as mindfulness, deep breathing, or meditation, to manage emotional and physiological stressors.
  - Chronic stress may impact metabolic factors associated with kidney stone formation.

- **Application:**

Regular Practice: Establish a routine of regular stress-reducing activities to promote emotional well-being.

Integration into Daily Life: Integrate stress reduction techniques into daily life, especially during challenging periods.

Smoking Cessation: Clearing the Renal Pathways

- **Impact of Smoking on Renal Health:**
- Quit smoking to mitigate the adverse effects of tobacco on renal function.
- Smoking is associated with an increased risk of kidney stone formation and exacerbates other kidney-related conditions.

- **Application:**

Smoking Cessation Programs: Seek support from smoking cessation programs or healthcare professionals to quit smoking.

Commitment to Health: Understand and communicate the profound impact that smoking cessation has on overall health, including renal resilience.

Alcohol Moderation: Balancing Choices

- **Reducing Alcohol Consumption:**

- Moderation in alcohol consumption is advisable, as excessive alcohol intake can contribute to dehydration and increase the risk of stone formation.

- Alcohol can also impact uric acid levels, affecting the formation of uric acid stones.

- **Application:**

Awareness of Limits: Be aware of recommended limits for alcohol consumption and strive to stay within those boundaries.

Hydration Focus: If consuming alcohol, balance it with adequate hydration to offset its potential dehydrating effects.

Environmental Considerations: Hydration Beyond Diet

- **Climate and Hydration:**

- Adjust hydration practices based on environmental factors, such as climate and temperature.

- Hot and dry climates may necessitate increased water intake to counteract dehydration and minimize stone-forming conditions.

- **Application:**

Hydration Awareness: Be mindful of environmental conditions and adapt water intake accordingly.

Fluid-Rich Foods: Incorporate fluid-rich foods, such as fruits and vegetables, into the diet for additional hydration.

Medication Adherence: Consistent Support for Renal Health

- **Adherence to Prescribed Medications:**

- Consistently follow prescribed medication regimens as advised by healthcare professionals.

- Medications, such as those for pain management or stone prevention, play a crucial role in supporting renal health.

- **Application:**

Communication with Healthcare Providers:

Communicate openly with healthcare providers about any concerns or side effects related to medications.

Timely Refills: Ensure timely refills and adhere to medication schedules for optimal effectiveness.

Regular Health Check-ups: Monitoring Renal Vitality

- **Periodic Renal Evaluations:**
- Schedule regular check-ups with healthcare professionals to monitor renal health and address any emerging concerns.
- Periodic assessments may include urine tests, blood tests, and imaging studies to assess kidney function and stone-related factors.

- **Application:**

Proactive Healthcare: Take a proactive approach to health by attending regular check-ups, even in the absence of apparent symptoms.

Open Dialogue with Healthcare Providers: Foster open communication with healthcare providers to address any renal health queries or changes in health status.

Education and Awareness: Empowering Renal Advocacy

- **Understanding Personal Risk Factors:**

- Educate yourself about personal risk factors for kidney stone formation and recurrence.

- Awareness empowers individuals to make informed lifestyle choices that align with their unique health needs.

- **Application:**

Continuous Learning: Stay informed about advancements in renal health and kidney stone prevention.

Community Engagement: Contribute to the community's understanding of kidney stone prevention through education and awareness initiatives.

Social Support Networks: Building Resilient Foundations

- **Family and Community Involvement:**

- Cultivate social support networks, involving family, friends, and communities, to provide emotional support and encouragement.

- Social connections contribute to overall well-being and may help individuals cope with the challenges of kidney stone management.

- **Application:**

Open Communication: Share experiences and concerns with loved ones, fostering an environment of understanding and support.

Community Engagement: Participate in support groups or online communities where individuals facing similar challenges can exchange insights and encouragement.

Embarking on the path of kidney stone prevention and renal resilience involves a holistic integration of lifestyle modifications. By addressing physical activity, stress management, environmental considerations, and other aspects of daily life, individuals can not only reduce the risk of kidney stone formation but also cultivate a foundation of well-being that extends beyond renal health. This chapter serves as a guide

Physical Activity and Kidney Health

In the intricate tapestry of human health, physical activity emerges as a powerful brushstroke, painting vibrant hues of well-being across various bodily systems. This section explores the symbiotic relationship between physical activity and kidney health, shedding light on how regular exercise becomes a cornerstone for the prevention of kidney stones and the promotion of overall renal resilience.

Metabolic Harmony: Exercise as a Catalyst

- **Optimizing Metabolic Function:**
- Regular physical activity contributes to the optimization of metabolic processes, fostering a harmonious interplay of factors that support kidney health.

- Exercise aids in weight management, blood pressure regulation, and glucose control, all of which are pivotal for renal well-being.

- **Application:**

Cardiovascular Exercise: Engage in aerobic activities, such as walking, running, cycling, or swimming, to enhance cardiovascular health and metabolic function.

Consistent Exercise Routine: Establish a consistent exercise routine, incorporating both aerobic and strength-training exercises, for comprehensive metabolic benefits.

Weight Management: Lightening the Load on the Kidneys

- **Maintaining a Healthy Weight:**

- Regular physical activity plays a vital role in weight management, reducing the risk factors associated with kidney stone formation.

- Excess body weight can contribute to metabolic changes that increase the likelihood of stone development.

- **Application:**

Caloric Balance: Combine exercise with a balanced diet to achieve and maintain a healthy weight.

Consultation with Fitness Professionals: Seek guidance from fitness professionals or healthcare providers to tailor exercise programs that align with weight management goals.

Blood Pressure Regulation: Exercise as a Natural Antihypertensive

- **Blood Pressure Control:**

- Physical activity acts as a natural antihypertensive, helping regulate blood pressure levels.

- Controlled blood pressure is essential for preserving renal blood flow and minimizing stress on the kidneys.

- **Application:**

Aerobic Exercise Benefits: Incorporate regular aerobic exercise to enhance cardiovascular health and contribute to blood pressure regulation.

Monitoring Blood Pressure: Regularly monitor blood pressure and consult healthcare professionals for guidance on exercise intensity and duration.

Enhanced Blood Flow: Nourishing the Kidneys

- **Improved Renal Blood Flow:**

  - Exercise promotes enhanced blood flow throughout the body, including to the kidneys.
  - Adequate blood flow is crucial for the kidneys to efficiently filter waste products and maintain optimal function.

- **Application:**

Cardiovascular Workouts: Engage in cardiovascular workouts that increase heart rate and promote blood circulation.

Consistency is Key: Regular, consistent exercise is essential for sustaining improved blood flow and supporting renal health.

Glucose Regulation: Exercise's Role in Metabolic Stability

- **Glucose Control:**

- Regular physical activity aids in glucose regulation, contributing to metabolic stability.

- Stable glucose levels are important for preventing conditions that can impact kidney function.

- **Application:**

Combining Aerobic and Strength Training:

Incorporate a mix of aerobic and strength-training exercises for comprehensive metabolic benefits.

Consistent Exercise Routine: Maintain a consistent exercise routine to support ongoing glucose control.

Prevention of Insulin Resistance: Breaking the Metabolic Chain

- **Mitigating Insulin Resistance:**

- Exercise plays a role in preventing insulin resistance, a condition linked to metabolic disorders and an increased risk of kidney stones.

- Insulin resistance can contribute to elevated levels of calcium and oxalate in the urine, promoting stone formation.

- **Application:**

Interval Training: Consider incorporating interval training into workouts, as it has been associated with improved insulin sensitivity.

Consultation with Healthcare Providers:
Individuals with metabolic conditions should consult healthcare providers for personalized exercise recommendations.

Urinary Dilution: Hydration Through Movement

- **Enhanced Urinary Dilution:**
- Physical activity promotes enhanced urinary dilution, an important factor in preventing the concentration of minerals that contribute to kidney stone formation.
- Improved urine dilution reduces the risk of mineral crystallization within the kidneys.

- **Application:**

Hydration During Exercise: Prioritize hydration before, during, and after physical activity to support urinary dilution.

Balancing Fluid Intake: Maintain a balance between fluid intake and loss during exercise, adjusting based on individual needs and environmental conditions.

Stress Reduction: Exercise as a Mental and Physical Tonic

- **Mind-Body Connection:**

- Exercise serves as a potent stress-reduction tool, benefiting both mental and physical well-being.

- Chronic stress may contribute to conditions that impact kidney health, making stress management crucial for renal resilience.

- **Application:**

Mindful Activities: Incorporate mindful activities, such as yoga or tai chi, into the exercise routine to promote stress reduction.

Consistent Practice: Establish a routine of regular exercise, as consistent physical activity has long-term benefits for stress management.

Adaptation to Environmental Factors: Kidneys in Motion

- **Adjustment to Climate and Conditions:**
 - Regular physical activity enables the body, including the kidneys, to adapt to varying environmental conditions.
 - Adaptation to climate influences hydration needs, supporting overall renal health.

- **Application:**

Hydration Awareness: Be mindful of environmental factors, adjusting hydration practices based on climate and temperature.

Fluid-Rich Foods: Incorporate fluid-rich foods into the diet, especially in conditions that may increase fluid loss through sweating.

Consultation and Customization: Tailoring Exercise for Kidney Health

- **Healthcare Professional Guidance:**

- Consult with healthcare professionals or fitness experts to customize exercise programs based on individual health needs.

- Individualized exercise plans consider factors such as age, existing health conditions, and personal fitness levels.

- **Application:**

Regular Health Check-ups: Prioritize regular health check-ups to assess overall health and receive guidance on exercise suitability.

Open Communication: Maintain open communication with healthcare providers to address any concerns or modifications needed in the exercise routine.

Embarking on a journey of physical activity for kidney health is a commitment to nurturing renal resilience through movement. By embracing exercise as a holistic tool that influences metabolic harmony, blood pressure regulation, and stress reduction, individuals can fortify their kidneys against the challenges posed by kidney stones, contributing to a vibrant tapestry of overall well-being.

Stress Reduction Techniques

In the hustle and bustle of modern life, stress has become an unwelcome companion, affecting not only our mental well-being but also influencing the intricate dance of our physiological systems. This section explores a repertoire of stress reduction techniques, offering a guide to cultivate inner harmony, enhance resilience, and mitigate the potential impact of stress on both mental and physical health.

Mindfulness Meditation: Anchoring in the Present

- **Mindful Awareness Practices:**

- Mindfulness meditation involves bringing attention to the present moment, fostering a non-judgmental awareness of thoughts and sensations.

- Mindfulness helps break the cycle of worry and rumination, promoting a sense of calm and clarity.

- **Application:**

Guided Meditations: Utilize guided mindfulness meditations, available through apps or online resources, to assist in cultivating a mindful practice.

Regular Practice: Dedicate a few minutes each day to mindfulness meditation, gradually extending the duration as comfort and familiarity grow.

Deep Breathing Exercises: Harnessing the Breath's Calming Power

- **Diaphragmatic Breathing:**

- Deep breathing exercises, focusing on diaphragmatic breathing, engage the body's relaxation response.

- Controlled, slow breaths can lower stress hormones and induce a sense of calm.

- **Application:**

4-7-8 Breathing: Inhale for a count of 4, hold for 7 counts, and exhale for 8 counts. Repeat several times.

Integration into Daily Routine: Practice deep breathing during moments of stress or as a regular part of your daily routine for cumulative benefits.

Progressive Muscle Relaxation: Unwinding Tension

- **Systematic Muscle Tension Release:**

- Progressive muscle relaxation involves sequentially tensing and then releasing different muscle groups, promoting physical and mental relaxation.

- This technique helps heighten awareness of bodily tension and teaches the body to release stress.

- **Application:**

Guided Sessions: Follow guided progressive muscle relaxation sessions available in audio recordings or apps.

Regular Practice: Dedicate time regularly to practice progressive muscle relaxation, especially during moments of heightened stress.

Yoga and Tai Chi: Moving Meditation for Body and Mind

- **Mindful Movement Practices:**

- Yoga and Tai Chi integrate mindful movement with breath, fostering a sense of tranquility and balance.

- These practices promote physical flexibility, strength, and mental relaxation.

- **Application:**

Beginner Classes: Start with beginner classes or online tutorials to explore the basics of yoga or Tai Chi.

Consistent Participation: Engage in these practices regularly, adapting them to your comfort level and preferences.

Nature Connection: Finding Serenity Outdoors

- **Outdoor Activities and Nature Immersion:**

- Spending time in nature has been linked to reduced stress levels and improved mood.

133

- Activities such as walking, hiking, or simply being in a natural setting can provide a therapeutic escape.

- **Application:**

Nature Walks: Incorporate short nature walks into your routine, taking time to observe the surroundings.
Mindful Observation: Practice mindful observation of nature's details, allowing your senses to engage fully.

Art and Creativity: Expressive Outlets for Stress Release

- **Artistic Expression:**

- Engaging in creative activities, such as drawing, painting, or crafting, provides an outlet for self-expression and stress release.
- The act of creation can be meditative, fostering a sense of accomplishment and joy.

- **Application:**

Art Journaling: Keep an art journal where you express emotions and thoughts through various artistic mediums.

Art Classes: Join art classes or workshops to explore new techniques and foster a sense of community.

Positive Affirmations: Cultivating a Positive Mindset

- **Empowering Self-Talk:**

- Positive affirmations involve repeating positive statements to oneself, promoting a shift toward a more optimistic mindset.

- Affirmations can counter negative thoughts, instilling a sense of self-compassion and resilience.

- **Application:**

Personalized Statements: Develop affirmations that resonate with your values and aspirations.

Daily Reflection: Incorporate affirmations into your daily routine, reciting them as part of a morning or bedtime ritual.

Journaling and Reflection: Processing Thoughts and Emotions

- **Written Expression:**

  - Keeping a journal allows for the expression of thoughts and emotions, providing a constructive way to process stressors.

  - Journaling promotes self-reflection and a deeper understanding of one's inner landscape.

- **Application:**

  Freewriting: Allow thoughts to flow freely onto paper without judgment or censorship.

  Gratitude Journaling: Include reflections on moments of gratitude to shift focus towards positive experiences.

Social Connections: Nurturing Supportive Relationships

- **Quality Relationships:**

  - Social connections act as a powerful buffer against stress, providing emotional support and a sense of belonging.

  - Sharing experiences and feelings with trusted friends or family members fosters a supportive environment.

- **Application:**

Regular Communication: Maintain regular communication with loved ones, even if it's through virtual means.

Social Activities: Engage in social activities that bring joy and a sense of connection.

Time Management and Boundaries: Creating Balance

- **Effective Time Allocation:**

- Managing time efficiently and setting boundaries helps prevent the accumulation of stressors.

- Prioritizing tasks and allocating time for self-care contribute to a sense of control and balance.

- **Application:**

Prioritization: Identify and prioritize tasks based on importance and deadlines.

Saying No: Learn to say no when necessary to avoid overcommitting and overwhelming yourself.

Embarking on a journey of stress reduction is an act of self-compassion and a commitment to nurturing mental and physical well-being. By integrating these techniques into daily life, individuals can cultivate resilience, foster inner harmony, and navigate life's challenges with a greater sense of ease.

CHAPTER 10: MEDICATION AND THERAPEUTIC APPROACHES

In the intricate landscape of kidney stone management, medication and therapeutic interventions stand as pivotal tools, offering targeted strategies to alleviate symptoms, prevent recurrence, and promote overall renal well-being. This chapter delves into the diverse array of medications and therapeutic approaches, providing insights into their applications, benefits, and considerations for individuals navigating the challenges posed by kidney stones.

Pain Management Medications: Easing the Path of Stone Passage

- **Nonsteroidal Anti-Inflammatory Drugs (NSAIDs):**
- NSAIDs, such as ibuprofen, can be effective in relieving pain associated with kidney stones by reducing inflammation.

- These medications are often prescribed to manage discomfort during stone passage.

- **Application:**

Prescription and OTC Options: Depending on the severity of pain, healthcare providers may recommend prescription-strength or over-the-counter NSAIDs.

Timing and Dosage: Follow healthcare provider recommendations regarding the timing and dosage of NSAIDs for optimal pain management.

Alpha Blockers: Facilitating Stone Passage

- **Relaxation of Ureter Muscles:**

- Alpha blockers, like tamsulosin, relax the muscles in the walls of the ureter, facilitating the passage of kidney stones.

- These medications are particularly beneficial for individuals with larger stones or stones causing significant discomfort.

Application:

Individualized Treatment Plans: Healthcare providers may tailor the use of alpha blockers based on the size and location of stones, as well as individual health factors.

Monitoring for Side Effects: Regular monitoring and communication with healthcare providers ensure the effective and safe use of alpha blockers.

Medications for Stone Prevention: Targeting Underlying Causes

- **Thiazide Diuretics:**

 - Thiazide diuretics, such as hydrochlorothiazide, may be prescribed to reduce the excretion of calcium in the urine, lowering the risk of calcium-based stones.

 - These medications are often used in individuals with a history of recurrent calcium stones.

- **Application:**

Regular Monitoring: Healthcare providers monitor urine and blood parameters to adjust thiazide diuretic dosage for optimal stone prevention.

Hydration Emphasis: Emphasize the importance of adequate hydration while taking thiazide diuretics to minimize the risk of dehydration-related stone formation.

Allopurinol: Managing Uric Acid Stones

Uric Acid Stone Prevention:
 - Allopurinol is prescribed to reduce the production of uric acid, a key factor in the formation of uric acid stones.
 - This medication is often recommended for individuals with a history of recurrent uric acid stones.

- **Application:**

Monitoring Uric Acid Levels: Regular monitoring of uric acid levels guides the adjustment of allopurinol dosage for optimal stone prevention.

Dietary Considerations: Healthcare providers may offer dietary recommendations to complement the effects of allopurinol in managing uric acid stones.

Dietary Supplements: Enhancing Stone Prevention Strategies

- **Calcium and Vitamin D Supplementation:**

- In some cases, healthcare providers may recommend calcium and vitamin D supplementation to prevent the formation of certain types of stones.

- Proper dosage and monitoring are essential to prevent imbalances that could contribute to stone formation.

- **Application:**

Individualized Recommendations: Healthcare providers tailor calcium and vitamin D supplementation based on individual needs, considering dietary intake and overall health.

Regular Monitoring: Periodic monitoring of calcium and vitamin D levels ensures the efficacy and safety of supplementation.

Extracorporeal Shock Wave Lithotripsy (ESWL): Non-Invasive Stone Fragmentation

- **Focused Shock Waves:**

 - ESWL involves the use of focused shock waves to break kidney stones into smaller fragments, facilitating their passage.

 - This non-invasive procedure is commonly employed for stones located in the kidney or upper ureter.

- **Application:**

Patient Selection: Healthcare providers assess the size, location, and composition of stones to determine if ESWL is a suitable option.

Post-Procedure Monitoring: Individuals undergo follow-up imaging to assess the effectiveness of stone fragmentation and to ensure the absence of complications.

Ureteroscopy: Direct Visualization and Stone Removal

- **Minimally Invasive Procedure:**

 - Ureteroscopy involves the insertion of a thin, flexible tube through the urethra and bladder to reach and remove stones in the ureter or kidney.

- This procedure is utilized for stones that may be challenging to treat with ESWL or are located in the lower ureter.

- **Application:**

Preoperative Assessment: Comprehensive imaging studies guide healthcare providers in planning and executing ureteroscopy.

Postoperative Care: Individuals receive postoperative care, including pain management and monitoring for potential complications.

Percutaneous Nephrolithotomy (PCNL): Surgical Stone Removal

Accessing Kidney Stones Through the Skin:

- PCNL involves creating a small incision through the skin to access and remove large or complex kidney stones.

- This surgical approach is reserved for cases where other methods may not be effective.

- **Application:**

Patient Selection: Healthcare providers carefully evaluate the size, location, and composition of stones to determine the appropriateness of PCNL.

Postoperative Recovery: Individuals undergo a recovery period with close monitoring for complications and follow-up imaging studies.

Dietary Modification Counseling: Tailoring Approaches for Prevention

- **Customized Nutritional Guidance:**

- Dietary modification counseling involves personalized recommendations to address specific factors contributing to stone formation.

- Healthcare providers work with individuals to develop dietary strategies that align with their unique needs.

- **Application:**

Stone Analysis: Recommendations are tailored based on the composition of stones, addressing factors such as calcium, oxalate, and fluid intake.

Long-Term Lifestyle Integration: Individuals receive ongoing support and education to incorporate dietary modifications into their long-term lifestyle.

Follow-up Care and Monitoring: Sustaining Kidney Health

- **Regular Check-ups and Imaging:**

- Individuals with a history of kidney stones undergo regular check-ups and imaging studies to monitor renal health and detect any emerging stone-related issues.

- Follow-up care ensures the effectiveness of preventive measures and timely intervention if needed.

- **Application:**

Communication with Healthcare Providers: Open communication with healthcare providers is vital for reporting any changes in symptoms or concerns.

Proactive Health Management: Regular follow-up appointments empower individuals to actively manage their kidney health and prevent recurrent stone formation.

Navigating the realm of kidney stone management involves a dynamic interplay of medications and therapeutic approaches, each tailored to address specific facets of stone formation, passage, and prevention.

Pharmaceutical Options for Stone Prevention

In the pursuit of kidney stone prevention, pharmaceutical interventions emerge as strategic allies, offering targeted solutions to mitigate the recurrence of stones and foster renal resilience. This section delves into the diverse array of pharmaceutical options, exploring their applications, mechanisms, and considerations for individuals seeking effective strategies to thwart the formation of kidney stones.

Thiazide Diuretics: Modulating Calcium Excretion

- **Objective:**
- Thiazide diuretics, such as hydrochlorothiazide, play a crucial role in preventing calcium-based kidney stones by reducing the excretion of calcium in the urine.

- **Mechanism:**

- Thiazides promote increased reabsorption of calcium in the kidneys' tubules, leading to decreased urinary calcium levels.

- **Application:**

Patient Selection: Healthcare providers consider thiazide diuretics for individuals with recurrent calcium-based stones.

Monitoring: Regular monitoring of urine and blood parameters guides adjustments in thiazide diuretic dosage to optimize stone prevention.

Potassium Citrate: Alkalizing Urine for Stone Deterrence

- **Objective:**

- Potassium citrate is employed to increase urinary pH, creating an environment less conducive to the formation of certain types of kidney stones, such as uric acid stones.

- **Mechanism:**

  - Citrate, a component of potassium citrate, binds with calcium in the urine, reducing the likelihood of crystal formation.

- **Application:**

  Uric Acid Stone Prevention: Potassium citrate is particularly beneficial for individuals prone to uric acid stone formation.

  Monitoring Acid-Base Balance: Healthcare providers monitor acid-base balance to ensure the optimal dosage of potassium citrate for stone prevention.

Allopurinol: Reducing Uric Acid Production

- **Objective:**

  - Allopurinol is prescribed to diminish the production of uric acid, a key contributor to the formation of uric acid stones.

- **Mechanism:**

  - Allopurinol inhibits the activity of xanthine oxidase, an enzyme involved in the production of uric acid.

- **Application:**

Uric Acid Stone Prevention: Allopurinol is particularly relevant for individuals with recurrent uric acid stones.

Regular Monitoring: Healthcare providers monitor uric acid levels, adjusting allopurinol dosage based on individual responses.

Calcium Supplements: Strategic Supplementation for Prevention

- **Objective:**

- Calcium supplements, when prescribed judiciously, can be part of a preventive strategy, especially for individuals with specific dietary considerations.

- **Mechanism:**

- Adequate calcium intake can help bind with oxalate in the intestines, reducing the absorption of oxalate and subsequently lowering the risk of calcium oxalate stone formation.

- **Application:**

Dietary Considerations: Calcium supplements are recommended based on individual dietary needs and in conjunction with dietary oxalate sources.

Monitoring Calcium Levels: Regular monitoring ensures that calcium supplementation aligns with individual requirements and doesn't contribute to hypercalcemia.

Antibiotics: Addressing Infections and Stone Formation

- **Objective:**

- Antibiotics may be prescribed to manage and prevent urinary tract infections (UTIs), which can contribute to the formation of certain types of kidney stones.

- **Mechanism:**

- By treating and preventing UTIs, antibiotics reduce the likelihood of infection-induced stone formation.

- **Application:**

Recurrent UTI Prevention: Antibiotics are considered for individuals prone to recurrent UTIs, which can be a risk factor for struvite stone formation. **Prophylactic Use**: In some cases, healthcare providers may prescribe prophylactic antibiotics to prevent UTIs in susceptible individuals.

Phosphate Binders: Mitigating Phosphate-Related Stone Formation

- **Objective:**
  - Phosphate binders may be recommended to individuals with specific metabolic conditions that predispose them to phosphate-based stone formation.

- **Mechanism:**
  - Phosphate binders bind with dietary phosphate in the intestines, preventing its absorption and subsequent excretion in the urine.

- **Application:**

Metabolic Considerations: Phosphate binders are prescribed based on the individual's metabolic profile and risk factors for stone formation.

Monitoring Phosphate Levels: Regular monitoring ensures that phosphate binders effectively address elevated phosphate levels without causing deficiencies.

Citrate Supplements: Enhancing Stone Prevention Strategies

- **Objective:**

  - Citrate supplements, such as potassium citrate, can be used to increase urinary citrate levels, which inhibit the formation of calcium-containing stones.

- **Mechanism:**

  - Citrate inhibits the crystallization of calcium oxalate and calcium phosphate, key components of some kidney stones.

- **Application:**

Calcium Oxalate and Calcium Phosphate Stone Prevention: Citrate supplements are particularly valuable for individuals prone to calcium oxalate and calcium phosphate stone formation.

Monitoring Citrate Levels: Regular monitoring ensures that citrate supplementation achieves the desired increase in urinary citrate levels.

Dietary Modification Counseling: Integrating Medications with Lifestyle Choices

- **Objective:**

- Dietary modification counseling involves personalized recommendations to complement pharmaceutical interventions, addressing specific dietary factors contributing to stone formation.

- **Mechanism:**

- Healthcare providers work with individuals to develop dietary strategies that align with their unique needs, optimizing the effects of medications.

- **Application:**

Customized Nutritional Guidance: Dietary modification counseling is tailored based on stone composition, metabolic factors, and individual preferences.

Long-Term Lifestyle Integration: Individuals receive ongoing support and education to incorporate dietary modifications and medications into their long-term lifestyle.

Regular Monitoring and Adjustments: Ensuring Optimal Effectiveness

- **Objective:**

- Regular monitoring of urine and blood parameters is essential to assess the effectiveness and safety of pharmaceutical interventions for kidney stone prevention.

- **Mechanism:**

- Monitoring allows healthcare providers to make adjustments in medication dosages based on individual responses, ensuring optimal stone prevention.

- **Application:**

Individualized Care Plans: Regular check-ups and laboratory tests form a crucial part of individualized care plans for kidney stone prevention.

Communication with Healthcare Providers: Open communication with healthcare providers is vital for reporting any changes in symptoms, concerns, or potential side effects.

Patient Education: Empowering Individuals in the Prevention Journey

- **Objective:**

- Patient education is integral to the success of pharmaceutical interventions, empowering individuals with knowledge about their medications, dietary choices, and the importance of adherence.

- **Mechanism:**

- Informed individuals are better equipped to actively participate in their kidney stone prevention journey, making informed decisions about medications and lifestyle choices.

- **Application:**

Understanding Medication Mechanisms: Patient education involves explaining the mechanisms of prescribed medications and their roles in stone prevention.

Lifestyle Integration: Educated individuals can integrate medications seamlessly into their daily routines and make lifestyle choices that align with stone prevention strategies.

Navigating the landscape of pharmaceutical options for kidney stone prevention requires a comprehensive understanding of individual health factors, stone composition, and metabolic considerations.

Emerging Therapies and Research

As the field of kidney stone management evolves, so does the quest for innovative therapies and cutting-edge research aimed at enhancing prevention, treatment, and overall renal health. This section delves into the realm of emerging therapies and ongoing research, offering a glimpse into the promising avenues that may shape the future of kidney stone care.

Nanotechnology in Stone Dissolution: Miniaturizing Solutions

- **Innovative Approach:**
- Nanotechnology holds promise in the development of miniature particles designed to target and dissolve kidney stones at a molecular level.

- **Mechanism:**
- Nano-sized agents may offer enhanced solubility and efficiency, potentially revolutionizing the dissolution of stones.

- **Research Progress:**
- Early-stage research explores the feasibility and safety of nanotechnology applications in kidney stone dissolution.

Microbiome Modulation: Harnessing Gut Health for Stone Prevention

- **Exploring Gut-Kidney Axis:**
- Research delves into the intricate relationship between the gut microbiome and kidney health, exploring ways to modulate the microbiome for stone prevention.

- **Mechanism:**
- Understanding how the gut microbiome influences the absorption of minerals and metabolites may unveil new strategies to prevent stone formation.

- **Research Progress:**
- Ongoing studies investigate the impact of probiotics, prebiotics, and dietary interventions on the gut microbiome and kidney stone risk.

Genetic Therapies for Inherited Stone Disorders: Targeting Root Causes

- **Precision Medicine Approach:**

- Advances in genetic research pave the way for targeted therapies addressing inherited conditions that predispose individuals to kidney stones.

- **Mechanism:**
- Gene therapies aim to correct or compensate for genetic mutations contributing to stone formation.

- **Research Progress:**
- Preliminary studies explore the feasibility and safety of genetic therapies for specific inherited stone disorders.

Biomarker Development: Early Detection and Personalized Care

- **Identification of Stone Risk Biomarkers:**
- Ongoing research seeks to identify biomarkers in blood or urine that can predict an individual's susceptibility to kidney stone formation.

- **Mechanism:**

- Biomarkers may offer insights into metabolic processes and genetic factors contributing to stone risk, enabling personalized preventive strategies.

- **Research Progress:**
- Exploratory studies focus on the discovery and validation of potential biomarkers for early detection and risk stratification.

Smart Implants for Stone Monitoring: Real-Time Insights

- **Innovative Implantable Devices:**
- Research explores the development of smart implants equipped with sensors to monitor urinary parameters in real-time.

- **Mechanism:**
- Implants may provide continuous data on factors such as pH, calcium levels, and crystal formation, offering dynamic insights into stone risk.

- **Research Progress:**

- Prototypes and feasibility studies assess the functionality, safety, and long-term viability of smart implants in kidney stone management.

Extracellular Vesicles in Stone Formation: Unveiling Cellular Communication

- **Cell-to-Cell Communication Focus:**
- Investigating the role of extracellular vesicles sheds light on how cells communicate in the context of kidney stone formation.

- **Mechanism:**
- Understanding the exchange of vesicles between cells may reveal novel pathways and targets for intervention.

- **Research Progress:**
- Early-stage research explores the complex interplay of extracellular vesicles in the context of renal physiology and stone development.

Drug Repurposing for Stone Prevention: Maximizing Therapeutic Potential

- **Utilizing Existing Medications:**
- Research explores the repurposing of existing medications, originally developed for other conditions, for their potential in kidney stone prevention.

- **Mechanism:**
- Drugs with known safety profiles may offer alternative preventive strategies by targeting specific pathways implicated in stone formation.

- **Research Progress:**
- Clinical trials investigate the efficacy and safety of repurposed drugs in diverse populations at risk of kidney stones.

Artificial Intelligence in Stone Analysis: Enhancing Precision

- **Computational Analysis of Stone Composition:**

- Integrating artificial intelligence (AI) into stone analysis may enhance the precision and efficiency of determining stone composition.

- **Mechanism:**
- AI algorithms may rapidly analyze imaging and spectroscopic data, aiding in accurate stone characterization.

- **Research Progress:**
- Pilot studies explore the integration of AI technologies in stone analysis, with the potential to streamline diagnostic processes.

Patient-Centered Digital Health Platforms: Empowering Individuals

- **Integrated Health Technologies:**
- Digital health platforms are designed to empower individuals in managing their kidney health, providing resources, tracking tools, and personalized guidance.

- **Mechanism:**

- These platforms may incorporate AI, telehealth, and educational resources to support individuals in adhering to preventive strategies.

- **Research Progress:**
 - Implementation studies assess the impact of digital health platforms on patient engagement, adherence, and outcomes in kidney stone management.

Comprehensive Lifestyle Intervention Trials: Holistic Approaches

- **Integrating Multifaceted Interventions:**
 - Research focuses on comprehensive lifestyle intervention trials that encompass dietary modifications, physical activity, and behavioral strategies.

- **Mechanism:**
 - Holistic approaches aim to address multiple facets of stone risk, offering personalized and sustainable preventive strategies.

- **Research Progress:**

- Longitudinal trials explore the effectiveness and feasibility of comprehensive lifestyle interventions in diverse populations at risk of kidney stones.

As the landscape of kidney stone management expands, emerging therapies and ongoing research illuminate new horizons for personalized, effective, and patient-centered care.

CHAPTER 11: HOLISTIC HEALING

In the realm of kidney stone management, embracing a holistic approach goes beyond conventional medical interventions. It extends into the interconnected realms of lifestyle, mindset, and spiritual well-being. This chapter explores the principles of holistic healing, providing a comprehensive guide for individuals seeking to foster not only physical resilience but also mental and spiritual harmony in their journey toward kidney health.

Mind-Body Connection: Cultivating Mental Resilience

- **Mindfulness Practices:**
 - Engage in mindfulness meditation and deep-breathing exercises to cultivate mental clarity, reduce stress, and enhance overall well-being.

- **Stress Reduction Techniques:**

- Explore progressive muscle relaxation, yoga, and tai chi to alleviate tension, promoting a harmonious mind-body connection.

Nutritional Wellness: Crafting Kidney Stone-Friendly Diets

- **Balanced Nutrition:**
- Adopt a diet rich in whole foods, emphasizing fruits, vegetables, and whole grains while moderating intake of high-oxalate and high-sodium foods.

- **Hydration Emphasis:**
- Prioritize hydration to maintain optimal urine volume, reducing the concentration of minerals that contribute to stone formation.

Physical Activity: Energizing the Body and Supporting Kidney Health

Regular Exercise:

- Incorporate regular physical activity into your routine, as it not only promotes overall health but also supports kidney function.

- **Targeted Exercises:**
- Explore exercises that enhance abdominal and pelvic muscle strength, potentially aiding in the prevention of kidney stone recurrence.

Holistic Therapies: Complementary Approaches for Well-Being

- **Acupuncture and Acupressure:**
- Consider acupuncture or acupressure sessions, which are believed to balance the body's energy and promote overall wellness.

- **Herbal Remedies:**
- Explore herbal supplements known for their potential to support kidney health, under the guidance of a qualified healthcare professional.

Emotional Well-Being: Nurturing the Heart and Soul

- **Expressive Arts:**
- Engage in creative outlets such as art, music, or writing as a means of self-expression and emotional release.

- **Mind-Body Practices:**
- Incorporate mind-body practices like journaling, positive affirmations, and guided imagery to foster emotional resilience.

Sleep Hygiene: Restorative Practices for Overall Wellness

- **Quality Sleep:**
- Prioritize good sleep hygiene, ensuring sufficient and restful sleep to support the body's natural healing processes.

- **Relaxation Techniques:**

- Practice relaxation techniques before bedtime, such as gentle stretching or meditation, to promote a calm and restful sleep.

Environmental Wellness: Creating a Supportive Surrounding

- **Nature Connection:**

- Spend time in nature to promote a sense of tranquility and connection with the natural world.

- **Decluttering Spaces:**

- Create a harmonious living environment by decluttering and organizing spaces, fostering a sense of calm.

Community Engagement: Building Supportive Connections

- **Support Networks:**

- Cultivate relationships with friends, family, or support groups to share experiences, seek guidance, and foster a sense of belonging.

- **Volunteerism and Giving Back:**
- Consider engaging in activities that contribute to the community, providing a sense of purpose and fulfillment.

Integrative Healthcare: Collaborative Approaches for Comprehensive Care

- **Collaboration with Healthcare Providers:**
- Explore integrative healthcare options, working in collaboration with healthcare providers who embrace both conventional and complementary therapies.

- **Personalized Care Plans:**
- Develop personalized care plans that consider individual preferences, beliefs, and the integration of holistic approaches into the overall treatment strategy.

Spiritual Well-Being: Nourishing the Soul

- **Meditation and Prayer:**
- Explore spiritual practices such as meditation, prayer, or mindfulness to nourish the soul and foster a sense of inner peace.

- **Reflective Practices:**
- Engage in reflective practices that align with personal beliefs, offering moments of introspection and connection with the divine.

Embracing holistic healing in the context of kidney stone management involves recognizing the intricate interplay between mind, body, and spirit.

Integrating Alternative Therapies

In the dynamic landscape of kidney stone management, the integration of alternative therapies provides a nuanced and holistic perspective that extends beyond traditional medical interventions. This section explores a spectrum of alternative therapies, offering insights into their potential roles in enhancing overall well-being and supporting individuals on their journey towards kidney health.

Herbal Medicine: Harnessing Nature's Remedies

- **Traditional Wisdom:**
- Explore the use of herbal remedies rooted in traditional medicine, known for their potential to support kidney health and prevent stone formation.

- **Cautious Exploration:**
- Engage in informed discussions with healthcare providers or herbalists to understand the potential benefits and risks associated with herbal supplements.

Traditional Chinese Medicine (TCM): Balancing Energy Flow

- **Acupuncture and Acupressure:**
- Consider acupuncture or acupressure sessions, integral components of TCM, believed to restore balance in the body's energy flow.

- **Chinese Herbal Medicine:**

- Explore formulations from Chinese herbal medicine, tailored to address specific imbalances that may contribute to kidney stone formation.

Ayurveda: Aligning with Natural Harmony

- **Dietary Guidance:**

- Embrace Ayurvedic dietary principles, emphasizing foods that align with your dosha to maintain balance and promote optimal digestion.

- **Herbal Supplements:**

- Explore Ayurvedic herbal formulations, such as those containing ingredients like Punarnava and Gokshura, believed to support kidney health.

Homeopathy: Tailoring Remedies to Individual Needs

- **Individualized Approaches:**

- Consult with a qualified homeopath to explore individualized homeopathic remedies, which aim to stimulate the body's natural healing mechanisms.

- **Supportive Measures:**
- Homeopathic practitioners may recommend remedies based on the totality of symptoms, addressing both physical and emotional aspects.

Mind-Body Practices: Aligning Mental and Physical Harmony

- **Yoga and Tai Chi:**
- Engage in mind-body practices like yoga or Tai Chi to enhance flexibility, reduce stress, and promote overall well-being.

- **Meditation and Guided Imagery:**
- Incorporate meditation or guided imagery to cultivate mental resilience, reduce anxiety, and foster a positive mindset.

Energy Healing Modalities: Balancing Vital Energies

- **Reiki and Energy Healing:**
- Explore energy healing modalities like Reiki to balance the body's vital energies, promoting a sense of relaxation and overall harmony.

- **Crystal Healing:**
- Consider crystal healing sessions, where specific crystals are believed to resonate with and support the energy centers related to kidney health.

Naturopathy: Holistic Wellness Practices

- **Dietary Counseling:**
- Consult with naturopathic practitioners for personalized dietary guidance, emphasizing whole foods and nutritional strategies to support kidney health.

- **Hydrotherapy and Detoxification:**

- Explore naturopathic approaches such as hydrotherapy and detoxification to enhance the body's natural elimination processes.

Aromatherapy: Scented Pathways to Relaxation

- **Essential Oils:**

- Incorporate aromatherapy using essential oils known for their calming properties, promoting relaxation and reducing stress.

- **Inhalation and Massage:**

- Enjoy the benefits of essential oils through inhalation or massage, creating a sensory experience that complements overall well-being.

Sound Therapy: Vibrational Healing

- **Tuning Forks and Singing Bowls:**

- Explore sound therapy using tuning forks or singing bowls, believed to have vibrational effects that support relaxation and balance.

- **Guided Sound Meditations:**

- Participate in guided sound meditations, which incorporate soothing sounds to enhance mental and emotional harmony.

Holistic Nutrition: Nourishing the Body and Soul

Whole Food Emphasis:

- Embrace holistic nutrition principles, emphasizing whole, nutrient-dense foods that support overall health and contribute to kidney stone prevention.

Individualized Plans:

- Work with holistic nutritionists to create individualized plans that consider dietary preferences, sensitivities, and specific needs for kidney health.

Caution and Collaboration:

- **Informed Decision-Making:**

- Approach alternative therapies with a spirit of curiosity and openness, but also exercise caution by seeking information and guidance from qualified healthcare professionals.

- **Collaboration with Conventional Care:**
- Foster collaboration between alternative therapies and conventional medical care, ensuring that all aspects of your health are considered in a comprehensive manner.

Integrating alternative therapies into kidney stone management is a personal and exploratory journey.

MindBody Connection in Kidney Health

The intricate interplay between the mind and body is a foundational aspect of overall health, and its significance becomes even more pronounced in the context of kidney health. This section explores the profound influence of the mind-body connection on renal well-being, emphasizing the importance of cultivating mental and emotional harmony to support kidney health and prevent the recurrence of stones.

Mindfulness Meditation: A Calming Influence

- **Stress Reduction:**
- Mindfulness meditation techniques, such as focused breathing or body scan exercises, can alleviate stress, which is a known contributor to kidney stone formation.

- **Cortisol Regulation:**
- Mindful practices have been associated with the regulation of cortisol, a stress hormone that, when elevated, may influence the formation of stones.

Stress and Kidney Health: Unraveling the Connection

- **Impact of Chronic Stress:**
- Prolonged exposure to chronic stress can contribute to imbalances in the body, potentially affecting factors like blood pressure and kidney function.

- **Inflammatory Response:**

- Stress-induced inflammation may impact the kidneys, emphasizing the need to manage stress for overall renal resilience.

Biofeedback and Relaxation Techniques: Harnessing Inner Control

- **Biofeedback Practices:**
- Biofeedback allows individuals to gain awareness and control over physiological processes, potentially aiding in stress reduction and blood pressure regulation.

- **Relaxation Response:**
- Engaging in relaxation techniques, such as progressive muscle relaxation or guided imagery, can elicit the relaxation response, positively influencing kidney function.

Emotional Well-Being and Kidney Health: An Interconnected Journey

- **Impact of Emotional States:**

- Emotional well-being, including feelings of joy, gratitude, and satisfaction, may contribute positively to kidney health by influencing factors such as blood flow and inflammation.

- **Negative Emotions and Kidney Stones:**
- Negative emotions, stress, and anxiety have been associated with an increased risk of kidney stone formation, highlighting the importance of emotional balance.

Cognitive Behavioral Therapy (CBT): Shaping Thought Patterns

- **Addressing Negative Thought Patterns:**
- CBT aims to identify and modify negative thought patterns and behaviors, providing tools to manage stress and enhance emotional well-being.

- **Behavioral Changes and Lifestyle:**
- By promoting positive behavioral changes, CBT may indirectly contribute to kidney stone prevention by addressing lifestyle factors.

Holistic Approaches to Mental Wellness: A Comprehensive View

• Incorporating Holistic Practices:
- Holistic approaches, such as yoga or Tai Chi, promote mental well-being through a combination of movement, breathwork, and mindfulness.

• Reducing Psychological Strain:
- The holistic nature of these practices addresses mental, physical, and emotional aspects, reducing psychological strain that may impact kidney health.

Psychoneuroimmunology: Understanding the Mind-Body-Immune Axis

• Interconnected Systems:
- Psychoneuroimmunology explores the connections between the mind, nervous system, and immune system, emphasizing the holistic impact on overall health.

- **Stress and Immune Function:**

- Chronic stress can influence immune function, potentially impacting the body's ability to manage inflammation and maintain kidney health.

Guided Imagery and Visualization: Harnessing the Power of the Mind

- **Positive Visualization:**

- Guided imagery techniques involve creating positive mental images, fostering a sense of well-being and resilience.

- **Relaxation and Reduced Anxiety:**

- Visualization can induce a state of relaxation, reducing anxiety and potentially positively affecting factors like blood pressure and stress hormones.

Lifestyle Modifications and Mental Well-Being: A Symbiotic Relationship

- **Healthy Lifestyle Choices:**

- Adopting a healthy lifestyle, including regular physical activity and balanced nutrition, positively influences both mental and kidney health.

- **Positive Feedback Loop:**
- The synergy between positive lifestyle choices and mental well-being creates a feedback loop, reinforcing overall resilience and supporting kidney health.

Patient Empowerment: Active Participation in Well-Being

- **Informed Decision-Making:**
- Empowering individuals to understand the mind-body connection fosters informed decision-making in managing stress, emotions, and overall well-being.

- **Collaboration with Healthcare Providers:**
- Collaboration between patients and healthcare providers facilitates comprehensive care that considers both medical interventions and holistic approaches to kidney health.

Understanding and nurturing the mind-body connection is an integral aspect of kidney health. This chapter serves as a guide for individuals seeking to embrace the interconnectedness of mental and physical well-being, fostering resilience and supporting the prevention of kidney stones through a holistic approach.

CHAPTER 12: LIVING WITH KIDNEY STONES: Practical Tips

Living with kidney stones requires a proactive and informed approach to manage symptoms, reduce the risk of recurrence, and enhance overall well-being. This chapter provides practical tips and strategies to empower individuals in navigating daily life with kidney stones, fostering resilience, and embracing a lifestyle conducive to renal health.

Hydration as a Daily Ritual:

Consistent Water Intake:
- Maintain adequate hydration by making water consumption a daily ritual. Aim for a sufficient intake of fluids throughout the day to promote urine dilution and reduce the risk of stone formation.

- **Lemon Water Benefits:**

- Consider adding a splash of lemon to your water, as citrate in lemon may help inhibit the formation of certain types of kidney stones.

Balanced Nutrition for Kidney Health:

- **Moderation of Oxalate-Rich Foods:**
- Be mindful of oxalate-rich foods such as spinach, nuts, and chocolate. Moderation can help manage oxalate levels in the urine.

- **Calcium-Rich Diet:**
- Include adequate calcium in your diet, either through dietary sources or supplements, as it can bind with oxalate in the intestines, reducing its absorption and subsequent excretion in the urine.

Mindful Dietary Choices:

- **Limiting Sodium Intake:**
- Limit sodium intake to support overall health and help manage blood pressure, which is essential for kidney health.

- **Protein Moderation:**

- Consume proteins in moderation, as excessive protein intake may contribute to certain types of kidney stones.

Regular Physical Activity:

- **Promoting Blood Flow:**

- Engage in regular physical activity to promote blood flow to the kidneys and overall cardiovascular health.

- **Targeted Exercises:**

- Include exercises that strengthen abdominal and pelvic muscles, potentially assisting in the prevention of kidney stone recurrence.

Stress Management Strategies:

- **Mindfulness Practices:**

- Incorporate mindfulness practices, such as meditation and deep-breathing exercises, to manage stress and reduce its impact on kidney health.

- **Hobbies and Relaxation Techniques:**
- Explore hobbies and relaxation techniques that bring joy and help alleviate stress, contributing to overall well-being.

Medication Adherence and Monitoring:

- **Timely Medication:**
- Adhere to prescribed medications as directed by healthcare providers to manage underlying conditions and prevent stone recurrence.

- **Regular Monitoring:**
- Schedule regular check-ups and follow-up appointments to monitor kidney function and make necessary adjustments to your treatment plan.

Bathroom Habits for Stone Prevention:

- **Frequent Urination:**

- Respond promptly to the urge to urinate to avoid concentrated urine, reducing the risk of crystal formation.

- **Proper Wiping Technique:**
- Adopt a gentle wiping technique after bowel movements to prevent irritation and potential stone formation.

Emergency Preparedness:

- **Pain Management Plan:**
- Have a pain management plan in place for sudden onset of kidney stone pain. Discuss this plan with healthcare providers and ensure access to prescribed pain medications.

- **Contact Information:**
- Keep a list of emergency contacts and healthcare providers readily available in case of severe pain or complications.

Support Networks:

- ## Connecting with Others:
- Join support groups or online communities to connect with others experiencing similar challenges. Sharing experiences and advice can provide valuable support.

- ## Family and Friends:
- Educate family and friends about kidney stones, helping them understand the condition and providing a supportive network.

Long-Term Lifestyle Integration:

- ## Gradual Changes:
- Implement lifestyle changes gradually to ensure long-term adherence. Sustainable habits contribute to ongoing kidney health.

- ## Adaptability:

- Be adaptable in your approach, making adjustments to your lifestyle as needed based on personal experiences and healthcare provider recommendations.

Living with kidney stones requires a multifaceted approach that combines dietary choices, hydration practices, stress management, and adherence to medical recommendations.

Everyday Coping Strategies

Living with kidney stones requires a thoughtful and proactive approach to daily life. This section explores practical coping strategies designed to help individuals manage symptoms, reduce the risk of recurrence, and maintain overall well-being while navigating the challenges of kidney stone management.

Hydration Habits: The Cornerstone of Kidney Health

- **Water, Your Daily Companion:**

- Develop a habit of carrying a reusable water bottle and sip water consistently throughout the day. Proper hydration helps dilute urine and prevent the concentration of minerals that lead to stone formation.

- **Infuse Flavor Mindfully:**
- Infuse your water with a splash of citrus fruits like lemon or lime. Citrate in citrus fruits may help inhibit certain types of kidney stones.

Mindful Nutrition: Crafting a Kidney-Friendly Diet

- **Balanced Choices:**
- Adopt a balanced diet rich in fruits, vegetables, whole grains, and lean proteins. Moderation in consuming oxalate-rich foods is crucial.

- **Calcium Considerations:**
- Include adequate calcium in your diet, either through foods or supplements, as it can bind with oxalates, reducing their absorption and subsequent excretion in the urine.

Portable Snack Kit: Smart Eating On the Go

- **Healthy Snacking:**

- Prepare a portable snack kit with kidney-friendly options like nuts, seeds, and fruits. Having nutritious snacks readily available ensures you make mindful choices even on busy days.

- **Plan Ahead:**

- Plan your meals and snacks, especially when away from home. Planning ahead helps you avoid foods that may contribute to stone formation and stick to your dietary goals.

Physical Activity: Energizing Your Body, Supporting Your Kidneys

- **Regular Movement:**

- Incorporate regular physical activity into your routine. Exercise promotes blood flow to the kidneys, supporting overall kidney health and cardiovascular well-being.

- **Targeted Exercises:**

- Include exercises that focus on strengthening abdominal and pelvic muscles. This can be beneficial in preventing kidney stone recurrence.

Stress Reduction Techniques: Cultivating Calmness for Kidney Health

- **Mindfulness Practices:**

- Engage in mindfulness practices such as meditation or deep-breathing exercises to manage stress. Chronic stress can impact kidney health, making stress reduction essential.

- **Quick Stress Busters:**

- Develop a list of quick stress-busting techniques for busy moments. Short walks, deep breaths, or positive affirmations can provide instant relief.

Medication Management: Adherence and Awareness

- **Timely Medication:**

- Adhere to prescribed medications as directed by healthcare providers. Consistent medication management is crucial for managing underlying conditions and preventing stone recurrence.

- **Medication Reminders:**

- Set reminders or use medication management apps to ensure you take your medications as scheduled. This helps maintain optimal treatment effectiveness.

Self-Care Rituals: Nurturing Your Well-Being

- **Restful Sleep:**

- Prioritize quality sleep as it plays a vital role in overall health. Establish a calming bedtime routine to promote restful sleep.

- **Pampering Practices:**

- Incorporate self-care into your routine, whether it's enjoying a warm bath, practicing aromatherapy, or engaging in activities that bring joy and relaxation.

Communication and Education: Empowering Yourself and Others

- **Open Dialogue:**
- Communicate openly with healthcare providers about your experiences and concerns. A transparent dialogue ensures you receive the necessary support and adjustments to your care plan.

- **Educate Loved Ones:**
- Share information about kidney stones with family and friends. Educated and supportive loved ones can play a crucial role in your journey.

Portable Comfort: Creating a Stone-Friendly Toolkit

- **Pain Management Essentials:**

- Assemble a portable toolkit with pain management essentials, including prescribed medications, a heating pad, and any comfort items that bring relief during painful episodes.

- **Emergency Contact List:**
  - Keep a list of emergency contacts and healthcare providers in your toolkit for easy access during unexpected situations.

Celebrate Progress: Acknowledging Your Resilience

- **Small Wins Matter:**
  - Acknowledge and celebrate your achievements and progress, no matter how small. Recognizing your resilience fosters a positive mindset and motivation to continue your journey.

Everyday coping strategies are essential for navigating life with kidney stones.

Navigating Social and Emotional Challenges

Living with kidney stones not only brings physical challenges but also social and emotional complexities. This section delves into strategies for navigating these aspects, providing insights and practical tips to build resilience and foster a supportive environment amidst the unique social and emotional challenges associated with kidney stone management.

Open Communication: Bridging the Gap

- **Family and Friends:**

  - Foster open communication with family and friends about your condition. Educate them on the challenges and nuances of living with kidney stones, helping to build understanding and support.

- **Workplace Discussions:**

  - If comfortable, consider having a conversation with your colleagues or supervisor about your condition. This can facilitate a more supportive work environment and understanding of any needed accommodations.

Dealing with Misunderstandings: Education as Empowerment

- **Myths and Misconceptions:**

- Be prepared to address myths and misconceptions about kidney stones. Providing accurate information empowers you and those around you to better understand the condition.

- **Educational Resources:**

- Share reliable resources with friends, family, and colleagues to offer a deeper insight into kidney stones and their impact on daily life.

Coping with Stigma: Embracing Your Journey

- **Self-Acceptance:**

- Embrace your journey with kidney stones. Understand that it's a medical condition, and there's no shame in seeking support or making necessary adjustments to accommodate your health needs.

- **Educate and Advocate:**

- Advocate for yourself by educating others. By sharing your experiences and needs, you contribute to breaking down stigma and fostering a more supportive community.

Emotional Support Networks: Building a Safety Net

- **Support Groups:**

- Seek out kidney stone support groups, either in-person or online. Connecting with individuals who share similar experiences can provide emotional support and valuable insights.

- **Therapy and Counseling:**

- Consider individual or group therapy to navigate the emotional challenges associated with chronic health conditions. Professional support can be instrumental in developing coping strategies.

Impact on Relationships: Nurturing Connections

- **Communication with Partners:**
- Communicate openly with your partner about the impact of kidney stones on your life. This transparency fosters understanding and strengthens the emotional connection.

- **Intimacy Discussions:**
- Discuss any challenges related to intimacy openly and seek solutions together. Maintaining open communication is essential for sustaining a healthy relationship.

Coping with Anxiety and Depression: Seeking Professional Help

- **Recognizing Mental Health Needs:**
- Be attentive to your mental health. If feelings of anxiety or depression arise, seek professional help from therapists or counselors who specialize in chronic health conditions.

- **Medication Consideration:**

- If necessary, consider discussing medication options with mental health professionals. They can provide insights into managing emotional challenges while taking into account your overall health.

Social Engagement Strategies: Balancing Social Life

- **Planning Ahead:**

- Plan social engagements with consideration for your health needs. Choose activities that align with your energy levels and potential dietary restrictions.

- **Educating Peers:**

- Educate friends and peers about your condition, ensuring they are aware of any dietary restrictions or potential triggers during social gatherings.

Coping with Flare-Ups: Preparing and Communicating

- **Emergency Plans:**

- Have an emergency plan in place for dealing with sudden flare-ups of kidney stone pain. Communicate this plan to close friends or family members who may need to provide support.

- **Educating Immediate Circles:**
- Make sure those in your immediate circles are aware of the signs of a flare-up and how they can assist or seek help if needed.

Celebrating Milestones: Acknowledging Progress

- **Small Victories:**
- Celebrate small milestones in your journey with kidney stones. Recognizing achievements, no matter how minor, contributes to a positive mindset and emotional well-being.

- **Gratitude Practice:**
- Develop a gratitude practice to focus on the positive aspects of your life. This can be a powerful tool for maintaining emotional resilience.

Collaborating with Healthcare Providers: A Unified Front

- **Shared Decision-Making:**
  - Collaborate closely with healthcare providers to address both physical and emotional aspects of kidney stone management. Shared decision-making ensures a comprehensive and holistic approach to your well-being.

Navigating social and emotional challenges is an integral part of managing life with kidney stones. This section serves as a guide, offering practical strategies and insights to build resilience, foster supportive relationships, and navigate the complexities of emotional well-being associated with chronic health conditions.

CHAPTER 13: PREVENTIVE MEASURES

Preventing the recurrence of kidney stones is a crucial aspect of long-term kidney health. This chapter explores comprehensive preventive measures, offering insights and actionable strategies to empower individuals in proactively managing their lifestyle, diet, and overall well-being to minimize the risk of future kidney stone formation.

Hydration Mastery: The Foundation of Prevention

- **Daily Water Goals:**
- Establish a daily hydration goal tailored to your individual needs. Consistent water intake is essential for diluting urine and preventing the concentration of minerals that lead to stone formation.

- **Monitoring Urine Color:**

- Use urine color as a simple indicator of hydration. Aim for light yellow urine, signifying proper hydration.

Dietary Choices: Crafting a Stone-Resistant Diet

- **Oxalate Management:**
- Moderate the intake of high-oxalate foods such as spinach, beets, and nuts. Understanding and managing oxalate levels in your diet can contribute to stone prevention.

- **Calcium Inclusion:**
- Include adequate calcium in your diet, either through dietary sources or supplements. Balanced calcium levels help bind with oxalates, reducing their absorption.

Sodium Consciousness: Balancing Salt Intake

- **Limiting Sodium:**
- Keep sodium intake in check, as excessive salt can contribute to calcium excretion in the urine. Opt for fresh, whole foods and minimize the use of processed and salty foods.

- **Reading Labels:**

- Read food labels carefully to identify hidden sources of sodium in packaged products. Being mindful of sodium content supports overall kidney health.

Maintain a Healthy Weight: Striving for Balance

- **Body Mass Index (BMI):**

- Aim for a healthy BMI by adopting a balanced diet and regular physical activity. Maintaining a healthy weight contributes to optimal kidney function and reduces the risk of stone formation.

- **Consulting with Nutritionists:**

- Seek guidance from nutritionists to create personalized dietary plans that align with your weight management goals and kidney health.

Regular Physical Activity: Promoting Kidney Wellness

- **Cardiovascular Exercises:**

- Engage in regular cardiovascular exercises to promote blood flow to the kidneys. Activities such as walking, jogging, or swimming contribute to overall kidney health.

- **Strength Training:**
- Include strength training exercises to enhance muscle tone, especially focusing on abdominal and pelvic muscles to support kidney function.

Regular Monitoring: Keeping Tabs on Kidney Health

- **Periodic Check-ups:**
- Schedule regular check-ups with healthcare providers to monitor kidney function. Routine assessments help identify any changes early on and allow for timely interventions.

- **Urine Analysis:**
- Undergo periodic urine analysis to assess mineral levels and identify potential risk factors for kidney stone

formation. Monitoring urine composition is crucial for preventive measures.

Medication Adherence: Following the Prescribed Plan

- **Timely Medication:**

- Adhere to prescribed medications as directed by healthcare providers. Medications may include those to manage underlying conditions or specific drugs to prevent stone formation.

- **Follow-up Appointments:**

- Attend scheduled follow-up appointments to assess the effectiveness of medications and make necessary adjustments to your treatment plan.

Dietary Supplements: Tailored Support

- **Supplement Consultation:**

- Consult with healthcare providers or nutritionists to determine if dietary supplements are necessary. Vitamin

D or citrate supplements may be recommended based on individual needs.

- **Calcium and Vitamin D Balance:**
  - Ensure a balanced intake of calcium and vitamin D, as these play crucial roles in bone health and may impact kidney stone risk.

Lifestyle Adjustments: Holistic Well-Being

- **Stress Management:**
  - Incorporate stress management techniques into your routine. Chronic stress can impact kidney health, making stress reduction an integral part of preventive measures.

- **Quality Sleep:**
  - Prioritize quality sleep, aiming for 7-9 hours per night. Quality sleep supports overall health and contributes to kidney resilience.

Patient Education: Empowering Through Knowledge

- **Understanding Triggers:**
- Educate yourself about specific triggers that may contribute to kidney stone formation. Understanding your unique risk factors enables you to make informed choices.

- **Lifestyle Integration:**
- Integrate preventive measures into your daily life gradually. Sustainable lifestyle changes contribute to long-term kidney health.

Preventive measures are key to minimizing the risk of kidney stone recurrence.

LongTerm Strategies for Stone Prevention

Long-term kidney stone prevention involves adopting holistic strategies that address various aspects of lifestyle, diet, and overall well-being. This section explores comprehensive and sustainable measures aimed at minimizing the risk of kidney stone recurrence, fostering renal health, and empowering individuals to take control of their long-term stone prevention journey.

Hydration Habits: A Lifelong Commitment

- **Daily Water Goals:**
- Make adequate hydration a lifelong commitment. Establish and maintain daily water intake goals to ensure consistent urine dilution and prevent mineral concentration.

- **Hydration Awareness:**
- Stay mindful of your hydration needs, adjusting them based on factors like climate, physical activity, and individual health conditions.

Dietary Choices: Crafting a Kidney-Friendly Lifestyle

- **Ongoing Oxalate Management:**
- Continue to moderate the intake of high-oxalate foods as part of your daily dietary choices. Consistency

in oxalate management contributes to sustained kidney stone prevention.

- **Calcium Inclusion:**

- Maintain a balanced intake of calcium-rich foods or supplements, as advised by healthcare providers. This ongoing practice supports the binding of oxalates in the intestines.

Sodium Consciousness: A Lifetime of Mindful Eating

- **Lifelong Sodium Monitoring:**

- Keep a watchful eye on sodium intake throughout your life. Choosing fresh, whole foods and adopting a habit of reading food labels contribute to a sodium-conscious lifestyle.

- **Educating Future Generations:**

- Share your knowledge and habits with family members, especially younger generations, to foster a culture of mindful eating and sodium awareness.

Weight Management: A Continuous Journey

- **Sustainable Lifestyle Choices:**

- View weight management as a continuous journey rather than a short-term goal. Adopt sustainable lifestyle choices that contribute to maintaining a healthy weight throughout your life.

- **Regular Health Assessments:**

- Schedule periodic health assessments to monitor weight, body mass index (BMI), and overall well-being. This ongoing vigilance supports long-term kidney health.

Physical Activity: A Lifetime Commitment to Wellness

- **Integrated Exercise Routine:**

- Integrate regular physical activity into your daily life. Choose activities that you enjoy and can sustain over the long term to promote overall kidney wellness.

- **Adaptable Exercise Plans:**

- Adjust your exercise routine as needed with age and changing health conditions. Adaptability ensures that physical activity remains a lifelong commitment.

Periodic Health Check-ups: Lifelong Monitoring

- **Regular Kidney Function Assessments:**
- Continue to prioritize regular check-ups with healthcare providers for ongoing monitoring of kidney function. Timely assessments help identify and address any emerging issues.

- **Urine Analysis:**
- Periodic urine analysis remains crucial for understanding your unique risk factors and making informed adjustments to preventive measures.

Medication Adherence: Consistent Management

- **Long-Term Medication Plans:**
- Adhere to prescribed medications consistently, following the long-term plan outlined by healthcare providers. This commitment plays a vital role in

managing underlying conditions and preventing stone recurrence.

- **Routine Medication Reviews:**
  - Schedule routine reviews of medication plans with healthcare providers to ensure continued effectiveness and make any necessary adjustments.

Holistic Lifestyle Adjustments: Lifetime Well-Being

- **Stress Management as a Lifestyle:**
  - Cultivate stress management techniques as an integral part of your lifestyle. Incorporate practices such as mindfulness, meditation, or relaxation exercises into your daily routine.

- **Quality Sleep Throughout Life:**
  - Prioritize quality sleep as a lifelong commitment. Consistent, restful sleep contributes to overall well-being and supports kidney resilience.

Patient Education: Empowering for a Lifetime

- **Continuous Learning:**

- Stay informed about advancements in kidney stone research and prevention. Lifelong learning empowers you to make informed decisions about your health.

- **Educating Others:**

- Share your knowledge and experiences with others. Act as a resource for family, friends, and community members, contributing to a culture of kidney health awareness.

Family Health Legacy: Passing Down Prevention

- **Multigenerational Awareness:**

- Instill kidney stone prevention awareness in your family. Pass down knowledge and healthy habits to future generations, creating a lasting legacy of family well-being.

Long-term strategies for kidney stone prevention require a commitment to sustained lifestyle choices and ongoing awareness.

Creating a Personalized Prevention Plan

Crafting a personalized kidney stone prevention plan is a proactive and empowering step towards long-term renal health. This section explores the essential elements of creating a customized prevention strategy, considering individual health factors, lifestyle choices, and medical history to minimize the risk of kidney stone recurrence.

Comprehensive Health Assessment: Understanding Your Unique Profile

- **Medical History Review:**
  - Begin by conducting a thorough review of your medical history. Consider factors such as past kidney stone episodes, family history, and any underlying health conditions.

- **Current Health Evaluation:**
  - Assess your current health status, including kidney function, through medical examinations and relevant

diagnostic tests. This baseline evaluation informs the development of a personalized prevention plan.

Consultation with Healthcare Providers: Partnering for Optimal Care

- **Nephrologist or Urologist Collaboration:**
  - Collaborate with a nephrologist or urologist specializing in kidney health. Their expertise ensures a focused and tailored approach to your prevention plan.

- **Multidisciplinary Team Involvement:**
  - Involve other healthcare professionals as needed, such as dietitians, nutritionists, and specialists in areas like endocrinology, to address specific aspects of your health contributing to stone formation.

Identifying Individual Risk Factors: Precision in Prevention

- **Type of Kidney Stones:**
  - Identify the specific type of kidney stones you've experienced. Different stones may require unique

preventive measures, such as dietary adjustments or specific medications.

- **Contributing Health Factors:**
- Consider factors such as metabolic disorders, urinary tract abnormalities, or genetic predispositions. Understanding these factors helps tailor prevention strategies to your unique health profile.

Lifestyle Assessment: Integrating Healthy Habits

- **Dietary Habits:**
- Evaluate your current dietary habits, including preferences, restrictions, and any specific dietary patterns. This assessment guides the development of a kidney stone-friendly diet.

- **Physical Activity Profile:**
- Assess your current level of physical activity and identify activities you enjoy. Tailor an exercise plan that aligns with your preferences and supports kidney health.

Dietary Customization: Tailoring Nutrition for Kidney Health

- **Oxalate Management:**
- Customize your diet to manage oxalate levels based on your specific tolerance. Some individuals may need stricter limitations on high-oxalate foods.

- **Calcium Intake Adjustment:**
- Adjust your calcium intake in consultation with healthcare providers. Tailoring calcium levels helps prevent oxalates from forming crystals in the kidneys.

Fluid Intake Strategy: Individualized Hydration Goals

- **Personalized Hydration Plan:**
- Determine your optimal daily fluid intake based on factors like body weight, climate, and activity levels. A personalized hydration plan ensures consistent urine dilution.

- **Monitoring Hydration:**

- Establish a system for monitoring your daily fluid intake, whether through a mobile app, journaling, or other methods. Consistency in hydration is key to kidney stone prevention.

Medication Plan: Adherence and Adjustment

- **Prescribed Medications:**
- If prescribed medications are part of your prevention plan, ensure strict adherence to the recommended schedule. Report any side effects or concerns promptly to healthcare providers.

- **Regular Medication Reviews:**
- Schedule periodic reviews of your medication plan to assess effectiveness and make necessary adjustments. Changes in health or lifestyle may warrant modifications to the preventive regimen.

Behavioral Strategies: Sustainable Lifestyle Changes

- **Stress Management Techniques:**

- Incorporate stress management techniques tailored to your preferences. Whether it's mindfulness, yoga, or other practices, choose methods that resonate with you for long-term adherence.

- **Behavioral Coaching:**
  - Consider working with behavioral coaches or therapists specializing in health-related behavior change. These professionals can provide guidance on making sustainable lifestyle adjustments.

Periodic Plan Reassessment: Adapting to Life Changes

- **Scheduled Reevaluation:**
  - Schedule regular reassessments of your prevention plan, especially during significant life changes, such as pregnancy, changes in work environment, or shifts in health status.

- **Adaptability and Flexibility:**
  - Embrace adaptability. Life circumstances may evolve, and your prevention plan should evolve with them.

Regular reassessment ensures ongoing relevance and effectiveness.

Educational Resources: Empowering Through Knowledge

- **Continuous Learning:**
- Stay informed about kidney health and advancements in preventive strategies. Continuously educate yourself on relevant topics to empower informed decision-making.

- **Educational Support:**
- Utilize educational resources provided by healthcare providers, reputable websites, and support groups. Knowledge is a powerful tool in maintaining kidney health.

Crafting a personalized kidney stone prevention plan involves a thoughtful blend of medical expertise, lifestyle considerations, and ongoing education. This chapter serves as a guide, emphasizing the importance of customization in preventing kidney stone recurrence and fostering lasting renal well-being.

CHAPTER 14: SUCCESS STORIES AND INSPIRATIONAL ACCOUNTS

In this chapter, we delve into narratives of resilience, strength, and triumph over the challenges of kidney stones. These success stories are not just tales of overcoming obstacles; they serve as beacons of inspiration for those on a similar journey. Each account is a testament to the human spirit's ability to persevere, adapt, and emerge stronger on the path to kidney health.

- **Sarah's Journey to Kidney Stone-Free Living:**
  - Sarah, facing recurrent kidney stones, embarked on a personalized prevention plan guided by her healthcare team. Through dietary adjustments, diligent hydration, and medication adherence, Sarah not only managed to prevent further stones but also experienced improved overall well-being. Her story showcases the transformative power of tailored preventive measures.

- **Mike's Resilience in the Face of Surgical Intervention:**

  - Mike's journey involved a series of surgical interventions to address persistent kidney stones. Despite the challenges, Mike approached each procedure with resilience and a positive mindset. His account illustrates the importance of adapting to different treatment modalities and maintaining optimism throughout the process.

- **Emma's Holistic Approach to Wellness:**

  - Emma embraced a holistic approach to kidney stone management, incorporating stress reduction techniques, regular physical activity, and a kidney-friendly diet. Her commitment to overall well-being not only contributed to kidney stone prevention but also enhanced her quality of life. Emma's story underscores the interconnectedness of lifestyle choices and kidney health.

- **Jason's Advocacy for Community Support:**

  - Jason, having navigated the complexities of kidney stones, became an advocate for community support. He initiated a local support group, providing a platform for individuals to share experiences, exchange information, and foster a sense of camaraderie. Jason's story highlights the empowering impact of community engagement in the kidney stone journey.

- **Maria's Journey to Empowerment Through Education:**
  - Maria, diagnosed with a rare type of kidney stone, embarked on a journey of education and empowerment. Through continuous learning, she collaborated with her healthcare team to develop a targeted prevention plan. Maria's story emphasizes the transformative power of knowledge in taking an active role in kidney stone management.

- **James' Successful Integration of Alternative Therapies:**
  - James, seeking a complementary approach to traditional medical interventions, integrated alternative therapies into his kidney stone management plan. Mind-body practices, herbal supplements, and dietary adjustments became integral parts of his preventive

strategy. James' account sheds light on the personalized nature of kidney stone management and the role of holistic approaches.

- **Lisa's Advocacy for Mental Health Support:**
- Lisa recognized the impact of kidney stones on her mental health and sought professional support. Through therapy and open communication with her support network, Lisa not only managed the emotional challenges but also developed resilience in facing the physical aspects of kidney stone management. Her story emphasizes the importance of mental well-being in holistic care.

- **Mark's Journey from Recurrence to Long-Term Prevention:**
- Mark, facing recurrent kidney stones, collaborated closely with his healthcare providers to identify underlying causes. With a tailored prevention plan addressing specific risk factors, Mark achieved long-term prevention. His journey exemplifies the significance of individualized care and persistence in achieving sustained kidney health.

- **Olivia's Story of Lifestyle Transformation:**

  - Olivia underwent a transformative lifestyle journey, adopting healthier habits and embracing a kidney stone-friendly diet. Her commitment to regular exercise, hydration, and balanced nutrition not only prevented further stones but also instilled a sense of vitality in her daily life. Olivia's story showcases the profound impact of lifestyle choices on kidney health.

- **David's Supportive Role in Family Well-Being:**

  - David, having experienced kidney stones, became a pillar of support for his family members facing similar challenges. His advocacy for open communication, shared experiences, and mutual encouragement created a resilient family support system. David's story illustrates the ripple effect of support within a close-knit community.

These success stories illuminate the diverse paths individuals have taken to triumph over kidney stones. Each narrative is a source of inspiration, offering insights into resilience, proactive management, and the transformative power of personalized approaches. As you read these accounts, may they instill hope, fortitude, and a sense of possibility on your own journey toward kidney health and well-being.

CHAPTER 15: SUPPORT NETWORKS AND RESOURCES

Building a strong support network and utilizing valuable resources is integral to the journey of managing kidney stones. This chapter delves into the importance of support systems and provides a comprehensive guide to the various resources available to individuals facing the challenges of kidney stone prevention, treatment, and overall well-being.

Peer Support Groups:

- In-Person and Online Communities:
- Explore local or online peer support groups where individuals share their experiences, insights, and coping strategies. Connecting with others who understand the journey can provide a sense of community and shared strength.

- **Anonymous Platforms:**

- Participate in anonymous forums or social media groups to discuss concerns, ask questions, and share victories. Anonymity can be empowering for those who may prefer a more private space.

Professional Support:

- **Nephrologists and Urologists:**
  - Cultivate a strong relationship with your nephrologist or urologist. Regular communication ensures personalized care, and these professionals can guide you through treatment options and preventive measures.

- **Nutritionists and Dietitians:**
  - Work closely with nutritionists or dietitians specializing in kidney health. Their expertise is invaluable in crafting a diet that supports your specific needs and minimizes the risk of stone recurrence.

Educational Resources:

- **Reputable Websites:**

- Explore reputable websites such as the National Kidney Foundation, Mayo Clinic, or the American Urological Association for reliable information on kidney stones. These sites often provide educational materials, articles, and guides.

- **Medical Journals and Publications:**
- Stay informed about the latest research by accessing medical journals and publications related to nephrology and urology. Knowledge from reputable sources can empower you in discussions with healthcare providers.

Mental Health Support:

- **Therapists and Counselors:**
- Consider therapy or counseling, especially if the emotional toll of managing kidney stones becomes challenging. Mental health professionals can provide coping strategies and support in navigating the emotional aspects of chronic health conditions.

- **Family and Friends:**

- Foster open communication with your family and friends about the emotional challenges you may face. Their understanding and support contribute significantly to your mental well-being.

Lifestyle and Wellness Resources:

- **Exercise Coaches or Physical Therapists:**
- Engage with exercise coaches or physical therapists who specialize in conditions affecting the urinary system. They can guide you in developing a safe and effective exercise routine tailored to your needs.

- **Stress Management Workshops:**
- Attend stress management workshops or classes, either in person or online. Learning effective stress reduction techniques contributes to your overall well-being and kidney health.

Medication Management Tools:

- **Medication Reminder Apps:**

- Use medication reminder apps to ensure consistent adherence to prescribed medications. These tools can be especially helpful for those with complex medication regimens.

- **Pharmacy Consultations:**
  - Schedule regular consultations with pharmacists to discuss your medication plan. Pharmacists can provide insights into potential interactions, side effects, and tips for managing medications effectively.

Patient Advocacy Organizations:

- **National Kidney Foundation (NKF):**
  - Explore the resources offered by patient advocacy organizations such as the National Kidney Foundation. These organizations often provide educational materials, support services, and opportunities for community engagement.

- **Kidney Stone Support Organizations:**
  - Connect with organizations specifically dedicated to kidney stone support. These groups may offer tailored

resources, webinars, and events focused on kidney stone management.

Government Health Agencies:

- **Centers for Disease Control and Prevention (CDC):**
  - Access information from government health agencies like the CDC for comprehensive insights into kidney health, preventive measures, and general well-being.

- **National Institute of Diabetes and Digestive and Kidney Diseases (NIDDK):**
  - Explore resources provided by the NIDDK, which conducts research and offers information on kidney diseases, including kidney stone prevention and treatment.

Financial Assistance Programs:

- **Health Insurance Guidance:**
  - Consult with health insurance representatives to understand coverage for kidney stone-related expenses.

Knowing your insurance benefits can alleviate financial stress.

- **Patient Assistance Programs:**
- Inquire about patient assistance programs offered by pharmaceutical companies or charitable organizations. These programs may provide financial support for medications or treatment costs.

Community Outreach Programs:

- **Local Health Clinics:**
- Explore community outreach programs offered by local health clinics. These programs may provide educational workshops, screenings, and resources for kidney health.

- **Community Events:**
- Attend community health events where professionals offer information on kidney health, preventive measures, and available support networks.

Building a robust support network and utilizing diverse resources contribute significantly to the holistic management of kidney stones.

Connecting with Others

Navigating the challenges of kidney stones can be a daunting task, but connecting with others who share similar experiences can be a source of strength, understanding, and shared wisdom. This section explores the significance of building connections within the kidney stone community and offers insights into the various ways individuals can connect with others on a similar journey.

Peer Support Groups:

- **Shared Experiences:**
 - Join local or online peer support groups where individuals facing kidney stones come together. Sharing experiences with those who understand the nuances of the journey can provide a sense of camaraderie and validation.

- **Anonymous Platforms:**

- Explore anonymous online forums or social media groups. Anonymity can be a comfort for those who prefer a more private space to discuss their challenges, seek advice, or share triumphs.

Online Communities:

- **Virtual Support Networks:**

- Engage in virtual communities dedicated to kidney stone warriors. Online platforms often host discussions, Q&A sessions, and provide a space for individuals to share their stories and insights.

- **Social Media Connections:**

- Connect with others on social media platforms using relevant hashtags or by joining kidney stone-related groups. Social media can serve as a dynamic space for exchanging information and fostering connections.

Local Support Networks:

- **In-Person Meetups:**

- Explore opportunities for in-person meetups with individuals in your local area. Meeting face-to-face can strengthen connections and provide a sense of community beyond the digital realm.

- **Hospital or Clinic Support Groups:**

- Inquire about support groups organized by hospitals or clinics specializing in urology or nephrology. These groups often bring together individuals dealing with kidney stone challenges.

Online Webinars and Events:

- **Educational Webinars:**

- Attend online webinars or virtual events hosted by kidney stone advocacy organizations. These events not only offer educational insights but also provide a platform for interaction and networking.

- **Patient Stories:**

- Listen to or share patient stories during webinars. Personal narratives can be inspiring and offer practical tips for managing different aspects of the kidney stone journey.

Family and Friends:

- **Open Communication:**
  - Foster open communication with your family and friends about your experiences. Their support can be a crucial pillar in your journey, and sharing insights with them creates a stronger support network.

- **Family Involvement:**
  - Encourage family members to attend educational sessions or support groups with you. Understanding the challenges and preventive measures can strengthen familial support.

Collaborative Healthcare Relationships:

- **Peer-to-Peer Networking:**
  - Connect with individuals recommended by your healthcare provider who have successfully managed

kidney stones. Peer-to-peer networking allows for shared experiences and practical advice.

- **Integrated Care Models:**

  - Explore healthcare models that integrate patients into their care team discussions. Collaborative care approaches can foster a sense of partnership in managing kidney stone-related challenges.

Social Media Advocacy:

- **Sharing Knowledge:**

  - Use social media platforms to share valuable resources and knowledge about kidney stones. Becoming an advocate in your online community can encourage dialogue and support.

- **Awareness Campaigns:**

  - Participate in or initiate awareness campaigns related to kidney stones. Raising awareness can not only contribute to community education but also create connections with those seeking information.

Community Outreach Programs:

- **Volunteer Opportunities:**
- Explore volunteer opportunities with kidney stone advocacy groups or community health organizations. Volunteering allows you to connect with a broader community while contributing to awareness and support initiatives.

- **Community Events:**
- Attend local health fairs or community events focused on kidney health. These gatherings provide opportunities to meet individuals with similar experiences and access valuable resources.

Creative Expression:

- **Blogs and Personal Websites:**
- Start a blog or personal website to share your kidney stone journey. Creative expression can be therapeutic for you and may resonate with others facing similar challenges.

- **Artistic Outlets:**

- Engage in artistic outlets such as writing, drawing, or music to express your experiences. Art has a unique way of connecting people and conveying shared emotions.

Seeking Professional Guidance:

- **Therapeutic Support:**

- Consider therapy or counseling for additional emotional support. Mental health professionals can provide coping strategies and a safe space to discuss the impact of kidney stones on your life.

- **Family Counseling:**

- If family dynamics are affected by kidney stone-related stress, consider family counseling. This can help improve communication and strengthen familial bonds.

Connecting with others in the kidney stone community is not only about seeking support but also about sharing insights, fostering awareness, and building a sense of solidarity.

Valuable Organizations and Websites

Accessing reliable information and finding supportive communities is crucial for individuals navigating the challenges of kidney stones. This section highlights valuable organizations and websites that offer a wealth of resources, educational materials, and supportive communities for those seeking information on kidney stone prevention, treatment, and overall well-being.

National Kidney Foundation (NKF):

Website: [National Kidney Foundation](https://www.kidney.org/)
Key Features:
  - Comprehensive information on kidney health and kidney stones.
  - Educational resources, articles, and guides for patients and caregivers.
  - Community engagement opportunities, including local events and support groups.

American Urological Association (AUA):

Website: [American Urological Association](https://www.auanet.org/)

Key Features:

- Professional resources and guidelines for urological conditions, including kidney stones.

- Patient education materials and information on treatment options.

National Institute of Diabetes and Digestive and Kidney Diseases (NIDDK):

Website: [NIDDK](https://www.niddk.nih.gov/)

Key Features:

- Research-based information on kidney stones and kidney disease.

- Clinical trials database for those interested in participating in research.

Mayo Clinic:

Website: [Mayo Clinic - Kidney Stones](https://www.mayoclinic.org/diseases-conditions/kidney-stones/)

Key Features:

- In-depth articles on kidney stones, their causes, symptoms, and treatments.
- Patient care and health information resources for comprehensive understanding.

Urology Care Foundation:

Website: [Urology Care Foundation](https://www.urologyhealth.org/)

Key Features:

- Patient-centered resources covering various urological conditions, including kidney stones.
- Educational materials, fact sheets, and videos for patients and caregivers.

American Association of Kidney Patients (AAKP):

Website: [AAKP](https://aakp.org/)
Key Features:
- Dedicated to kidney patient advocacy and education.
- Resources on living with kidney disease, including kidney stones.

KidneyStoners.org:

Website:
[KidneyStoners.org](http://www.kidneystoners.org/)
Key Features:
- Patient-driven website sharing personal experiences with kidney stones.
- Practical tips, forums, and a supportive community for individuals dealing with kidney stones.

MedicineNet - Kidney Stones:

Website: [MedicineNet - Kidney Stones](https://www.medicinenet.com/kidney_stones/article.htm)

Key Features:

- Clear and concise articles on kidney stones, symptoms, and treatments.

- Educational content for patients and those seeking general information.

Healthline - Kidney Stones:

Website: [Healthline - Kidney Stones](https://www.healthline.com/health/kidney-stones)

Key Features:

- Informational articles, slideshows, and videos on kidney stones.

- Lifestyle tips and insights into managing kidney stone symptoms.

Inspire - Kidney Stones Support Community:

Website: [Inspire - Kidney Stones](https://www.inspire.com/groups/kidney-stones/)

Key Features:

- Online community where individuals share experiences and support.

- Discussion forums covering various aspects of kidney stone management.

UpToDate - Patient Information: Kidney Stones:

Website: [UpToDate - Kidney Stones](https://www.uptodate.com/contents/kidney-stones-beyond-the-basics)

Key Features:

- Patient-friendly information on kidney stones, treatment options, and prevention.

- Reviewed by medical professionals for accuracy and reliability.

Reddit - Kidney Stones Community:

Website: [r/KidneyStones](https://www.reddit.com/r/KidneyStones/)

Key Features:

- User-driven discussions, personal experiences, and advice.
- An informal platform for connecting with others dealing with kidney stones.

These organizations and websites provide a wealth of information, support, and community for individuals facing kidney stone challenges. Whether seeking educational materials, connecting with a supportive community, or accessing the latest research, these resources can empower individuals to navigate their kidney stone journey with knowledge and resilience.

CONCLUSION

As we conclude this journey through the intricacies of kidney stones, it is essential to reflect on the wealth of knowledge gained and the empowering strategies presented. Managing kidney stones is a dynamic process, requiring a multifaceted approach that encompasses understanding, prevention, and resilient living. This chapter encapsulates the key takeaways and encourages a proactive mindset for sustained kidney health.

Knowledge Empowers:

- **Understanding the Enemy:**
 - Knowledge about the formation, types, and risk factors of kidney stones forms the foundation for effective prevention and management.

- **Diagnostic Awareness:**
 - Recognizing symptoms, seeking timely medical attention, and understanding diagnostic procedures

257

empower individuals to take control of their kidney health.

Prevention is Key:

- **Lifestyle Choices Matter:**
  - Embracing dietary modifications, staying hydrated, and adopting a kidney-friendly lifestyle are pivotal in preventing the recurrence of kidney stones.

- **Medication Adherence:**
  - Strict adherence to prescribed medications and consistent follow-up appointments with healthcare providers play a crucial role in long-term prevention.

Support is a Pillar:

- **Building a Support Network:**
  - Connecting with others facing similar challenges provides not only emotional support but also a platform for shared insights and coping strategies.

- **Leveraging Resources:**

- Valuable organizations, websites, and healthcare professionals serve as essential resources in the ongoing journey of kidney stone management.

Resilience in Everyday Living:

- **Holistic Approaches:**
- Incorporating holistic strategies, including stress management, physical activity, and dietary adjustments, contributes to overall well-being and kidney health.

- **Adaptable Lifestyle:**
- Recognizing the need for adaptability in lifestyle choices ensures that preventive measures remain relevant in the face of life's changes.

Patient-Centric Care:

- **Personalized Prevention Plans:**
- Crafting a prevention plan tailored to individual health profiles ensures a more effective and sustainable approach to kidney stone management.

- **Continuous Learning:**

- The journey doesn't end; it evolves. Continuous learning about emerging therapies, research, and holistic approaches contributes to ongoing kidney health.

Strength in Community:

- **Connecting Beyond the Pages:**

- Beyond the information presented in these chapters, the strength lies in the community – sharing experiences, supporting one another, and collectively advocating for kidney health.

In concluding this exploration into renal resilience, remember that managing kidney stones is not a solitary endeavor. It is a journey marked by knowledge, prevention, support, and resilience. May this guide serve as a compass, guiding you toward sustained kidney health and a future marked by well-being and vitality. Your journey continues, empowered and informed, as you navigate the path ahead with strength and determination.

Encouragement for Resilience and Continued Wellness

As you stand at the conclusion of this insightful exploration into kidney stone management, let these words be a beacon of encouragement, resilience, and optimism for the continued journey towards wellness. Navigating the challenges of kidney stones demands not just knowledge but also a spirit fortified with resilience. Here's a heartfelt encouragement for the path ahead:

1. Celebrate Your Progress:

 - Take a moment to acknowledge the strides you've made in understanding kidney stones and implementing preventive measures. Every step forward is a triumph.

2. Embrace Adaptability:

 - Life is dynamic, and so is your health journey. Embrace adaptability as a strength, allowing your prevention plan to evolve with the changes life presents.

3. Your Health is a Priority:

- Prioritize your health as an ongoing commitment. Regular check-ups, adherence to preventive measures, and self-care rituals contribute to your overall well-being.

4. Connect with Your Support System:

- Lean on your support network—family, friends, and fellow kidney stone warriors. Share your experiences, seek advice, and draw strength from the understanding and encouragement of others.

5. Be Kind to Yourself:

- Managing kidney stones can be challenging, both physically and emotionally. Be kind to yourself on this journey. Celebrate your victories, no matter how small, and recognize the effort you put into your well-being.

6. Embrace Holistic Well-Being:

- Wellness extends beyond the physical. Embrace holistic approaches to well-being, including stress management, a kidney-friendly diet, and activities that bring joy and relaxation.

7. Stay Informed and Curious:

- Knowledge is a powerful ally. Stay informed about advancements in kidney stone research and treatment options. Cultivate curiosity about your health, and don't hesitate to seek new information.

8. You Are Not Alone:

- Remember, you are not alone on this journey. Many individuals face similar challenges, and there's a wealth of support and understanding within the kidney stone community. Share your story, and let others share theirs.

9. Find Joy in Everyday Moments:

- Amidst the challenges, find joy in everyday moments. Whether it's a shared laugh, a moment of tranquility, or achieving a personal goal, these moments contribute to your overall well-being.

10. Resilience is Your Superpower:

- Your resilience is a superpower that propels you forward. Each day is an opportunity to overcome, adapt, and thrive. Trust in your inner strength and the resilience that resides within you.

As you continue on your path towards continued wellness, remember that the journey is not just about managing kidney stones—it's about embracing a life marked by vitality, connection, and well-being. Your commitment to resilience paves the way for a future filled with health, joy, and the unwavering belief in your ability to navigate the road ahead. Keep moving forward with determination, hope, and the knowledge that you are resilient beyond measure.

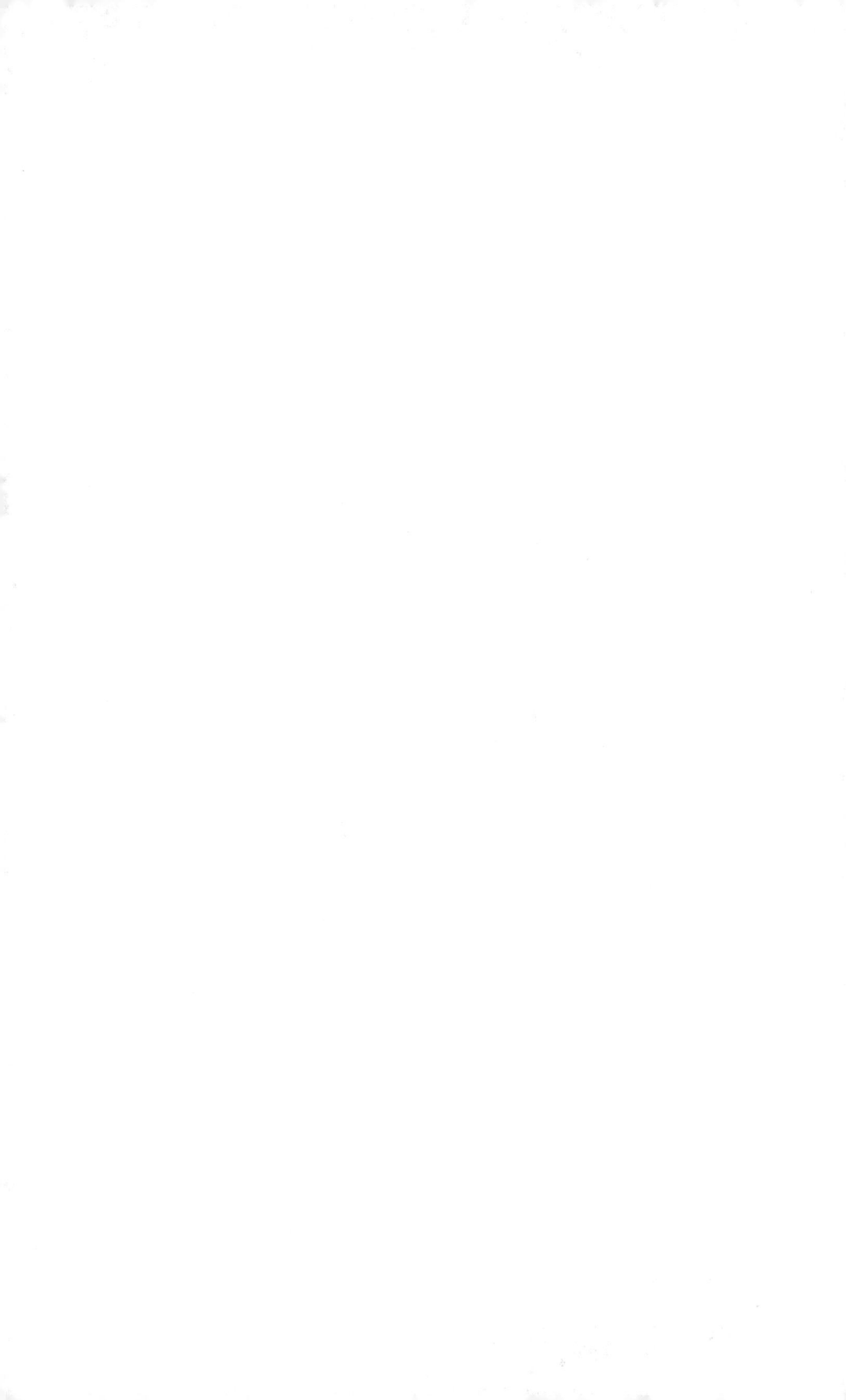